Myrcles

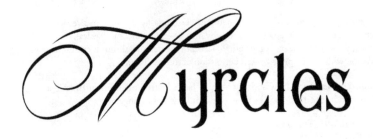

Myrcles

*A True Story of
Divine Intervention,
Hope and Inspiration*

CATHY ALVES DAVIS

NEW YORK

LONDON • NASHVILLE • MELBOURNE • VANCOUVER

Myrcles

A True Story of Divine Intervention, Hope and Inspiration

Published in New York, New York, by Morgan James Publishing. Morgan James is a trademark of Morgan James, LLC. www.MorganJamesPublishing.com

ISBN 9781631951336 paperback
ISBN 9781631951343 eBook
Library of Congress Control Number: 2020936191

Cover Photo by:
Matt Herriger,
used with permission

Edited by:
Susan Nelowet

Cover Design by:
Germancreative

Interior Design by:
Christopher Kirk
www.GFSstudio.com

Author Photo by:
Nikki Le

The names of some characters in this book have been changed or omitted for reasons of privacy. The author has related events and relationships in this book in good faith and with all due regard for personal and professional sensitivities.

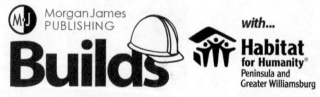

Morgan James is a proud partner of Habitat for Humanity Peninsula and Greater Williamsburg. Partners in building since 2006.

Get involved today! Visit
MorganJamesPublishing.com/giving-back

To my Heavenly Father;
Jesus, my Lord and Savoir;
my grandparents, Evelyn and Lyman;
my parents, Barbara and Frank;
my husband, George;
my children, Merritt, Blake, and Joanna;
and my grandchildren, Reagan, Drake, Lynleigh, Brynn, and Blakely

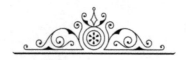

*"She believed she could,
so she did."*

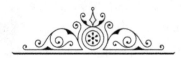

Contents

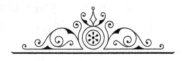

An Author's Prayer

*D*ear Heavenly Father, first and foremost, I want to thank you for all you have done for me. For redeeming me time and time again. For taking me out of the darkness of uncertainty and showing me the light. You saved me when no one else could, giving me new hope for a better future, and bestowing on me this awesome mission. When you spoke to me in 1998, in the midst of a cancer diagnosis, telling me I would go on to write a book of "hope and inspiration," I was filled with awe and anticipation. Even in those difficult days I believed in your message, and although I had never written a book before, I knew I could do it! After some years of healing, I began my challenging task. I wrote late at night, as you watched over my shoulder, and the words flowed easily as my story unfolded.

I could never praise you enough, Lord, for all you have done for me in never letting me down. And for always showing up in my life whenever I need you most.

Today, I sit at my desk as tears of joy pour down my cheeks and my spirit overflows with gratitude. The story you told me to tell all those years ago has gone on to help thousands of people. But you told me the book would give "hope and inspiration to countless others." I remembered your words and never for a moment doubted or forgot them. I did all I could, Lord, as one person to make that happen. My mission may have seemed impossible to others, but I believed in you. I know you can do the impossible so I simply stayed in faith.

It was no surprise to me when Morgan James Publishing, of New York City, decided to publish my book, making it available to bookstores everywhere. I know, too, you hand-selected them to enable me to share my story of faith, hope, and inspiration to the world. Now, Lord, just as you promised twenty-three years ago, as my life was in the balance and no one but you offered me any hope, Myrcles will go out and truly touch the lives of countless others!

I remain your faithful and loving servant here on Earth while hoping to always demonstrate "How Great Thou Art."

In Jesus precious name I pray,

Amen

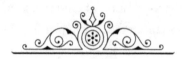

Introduction

I want you to know that God told me to write this book, telling me to do so with you in mind, knowing you'd need His loving care throughout your life, even more in times of sadness, struggles, marital problems, child rearing, job pressures, disappointments, betrayal, stress, financial woes, and especially when facing cancer.

In early 1998, as I lay on the CT scan table at Beth Israel Hospital in Boston, being scanned to see if my newly diagnosed aggressive stage III breast cancer had spread, God spoke to me, allowing me to know I would be fine, telling me that one day I would go on to write a book of hope and inspiration. At the time, I thought He was talking about surviving cancer. But in the twenty-three years that have followed, I've realized that He was talking about all the areas in a woman's life.

In my book you'll see how faith can take you over the mountains we all come up against in this lifetime. You'll read about the many miracles

God has provided me, not just in curing my cancer, but from the time I was a young girl, desperate to breathe from the affliction of asthma. I do not believe I am special or unique in being able to discern God's miracles. They are here for each one of us, right before our eyes, if only we see—if only we have *faith*, the foundation of everything I am about to tell you. "Now faith is the substance of things hoped for, the evidence of things not seen." (Hebrews 11: 1, KJV)

Throughout my life I have been touched and guided by Divine Intervention. I want to bring that message to you through the many scenes and incidents in this book. Many of you might consider my cure from cancer to be the most dramatic or important of the miracles, for understandable reasons, but I want to emphasize that *all* of God's interventions have been miracles, from a tiny bird landing on my hand early in life to the gift of helping ill and despairing friends later in life. My essential point is that *faith* allows us to perceive the fullness of God's enveloping love, in all of its minute or staggering glory.

As I began to write this book I expected to call it *Divine Intervention*, naturally enough. I soon learned, however, that hundreds of other books carry this title, and I didn't want my message of faith and hope to be lost in a crowded field. As with so many decisions I face, I placed the title of my book in prayer, knowing God would assist me in finding the perfect name. He did this by helping me realize, through my husband, that the name had been in front of me for some time already, actually on the front and back of my car. I hadn't made the connection until the day my husband called me from his office and said he had just had the thought, for no apparent reason, that "It's your license plate . . .'MYRCLE.'"

Nearly two decades ago, when personalized Breast Cancer plates were made available in our state, I knew I had to have one that said "Miracle." That would be my message, with the pink ribbon displayed proudly beside it, spreading hope and giving women food for thought as they saw it. But the license plate could accommodate only six characters, meaning I needed to brainstorm a creative way to say the word. Thus, *MYRCLES* was born, or "My Miracle" as I like to interpret it, adding the "s" to account for all the miracles I am about to describe. (To this day, my license plate, now a little bent and faded but still distinctive, continues to spark conversation wherever I go, allowing me to touch on my story of Divine Intervention.)

I have purposely left out my religious affiliation in this book. Religion is what we practice, often times due to the religion of our youth, giving us a means to exercise our belief system, while spirituality is something we choose for ourselves. There are many avenues of practicing our religious freedoms, recognizing that each religion is skeptical of the practices of the other, but spirituality goes far beyond religious practice; it is the spirit yearning for its true connection to our life source, the Almighty.

My fervent goal is to have this book speak to you wherever you are on your personal journey. You may already have deep and abiding faith and will read my story as affirmation. You may be facing troubled times in any number of ways and are looking for guidance or consolation—believe me, I have climbed many mountains' worth of trouble and have lived to tell about it. Or, you may be searching, wondering, just how do I come to faith, or how does faith find me, or just *what is it* about faith that I'm not understanding? Welcome to my story, a spirit-enhancing opportunity to see what it's all about.

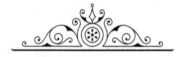

Section I
The Gift of Faith

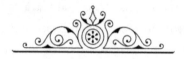

The Miracles Begin

He said to her, "Daughter, your faith has healed you.
Go in peace and be free from your suffering."
Mark 5:34

I could not tell you my story without telling you the whole story—
where I came from and what happened to me in my childhood:
happenings that shaped my life, giving me the Gift of Faith.

For me, home was a beautiful little seaside town called Duxbury,
Massachusetts, a picturesque place to live. I lived there with my parents,
Barbara and Frank Alves, and my two younger sisters, Holly and Nancy.
We grew up in the fifties and sixties on a street called Landing Road,
three houses up from the beach on the bayside.

I was a fair-skinned, blue-eyed blonde who smiled and laughed a lot,
a happy child. I never met a stranger, nor was I ever at a loss for words.

My parents were much like Lucille Ball and Desi Arnaz. My mother was a beauty with a quick wit, inherited from her father. My father was a handsome man who adored my mother, finding her humorous antics endearing and nicknaming her "Beautiful."

My maternal grandparents, Nana and Gaga as I called them, were a second set of parents to me, a wonderful couple, and I loved them dearly. They lived about a mile from our home. My grandmother, a small, redheaded woman, was on the quiet side with a sweet and loving personality. My grandfather was a fearless powerhouse, towering over my grandmother in stature. He was completely extroverted and easily captivated audiences with his animated story-telling ability. His most endearing quality, though, was being a friend to all!

My mother's younger brother, Uncle Donnie, lived with my grandparents, too. He'd contracted spinal meningitis as an infant in the thirties. By God's grace he was one of the first infants to survive that frightening illness back then, but the high fevers left him with a learning disability. He held many odd jobs in Duxbury during my growing up years, but his favorite was to hoist the flag up the pole in the center of town each day.

From the time I started school my bus route took me past my grandparent's home, where my grandmother stood at her window, throwing me a kiss and waving me on to my day of learning. As the years passed by, my school bus full of kids, along with the driver, waved back. Then we rounded the flagpole in the center of town, so close I could look down at my uncle from my seat on the bus, waving at him as he accomplished his task.

This idyllic setting provided a warm and loving environment for my childhood, and to this day I return to Duxbury every year for family reunions and spiritual and emotional renewal. However, my happy childhood had one big problem (as every family has problems) that couldn't be easily managed: I was diagnosed at an early age with asthma. In those days there was no magic bullet for asthmatics; we just suffered and gasped for air. An asthma attack feels like someone much larger than you sitting on your chest and holding a pillow over your mouth, causing you to panic and struggle for air, your heart beating faster and faster to the point of pounding fury. Sometimes in those days it was too much for children; their hearts simply gave out.

My attacks could go on for hours, chest heaving and coughing and strangling. Until the attack was finished, there was little anyone could do. Only ever so slowly did my breathing return to normal.

The attacks seemed always to come in the middle of the night. I would be dreaming that I was gasping for air, only to awaken to my very real nightmare! In my fear and breathless state it took all my strength to call out to my mother. Looking toward the hallway, I could see her bedroom light come on, and in a moment she was at my bedside, stroking my brow in an effort to calm my fears.

Then she would help me move downstairs to the green sofa, where it was cooler; together we'd get through another breathless night. Most of the time my mother never turned the downstairs lights on during these late night attacks. Instead, she relied on the moon's glow to fill the room with a heavenly aura.

She placed a pillow under my head as she began to talk softly, stroking me as she urged me to relax and work with my body. If the attack were severe I'd become disheartened, frightened, and panicked as my body fought for the air that wouldn't come. At that point my mother knew there was nothing humanly possible she could do for me—my wellbeing was out of her hands.

It was there in that holy room that my mother would tell me to go to Jesus, whispering, "Close your eyes, dear, and go to Him...He's come to help you, can you see Him as He walks toward you in His long, blue robe. He knows you are suffering. His healing hands reach out for you to heal you once again this night."

I was so weak, lying there exhausted and still gasping, but with my mother's sweet coaxing and whispers, I would finally relax enough to drift off to sleep. And just as she promised, Jesus came toward me, much like He's depicted in the Bible, wearing His magnificent blue robe, kindness written all over His face. I was always so grateful to see Him, knowing my suffering was over. I felt His presence communicate with me, not in words, but in a complete understanding of the peace he was conveying.

The mornings after these breathing attacks I would awake to a room transformed from heavenly incandescence to bright workaday sunlight. Seeing my eyes open, my mother would sit down beside me, my breathing thankfully back to normal. Even though I was very young, I could recount to her my experience with Jesus. Maybe at the time my mother thought I only dreamed of Him—but as my childhood progressed she witnessed Divine Intervention in my life so many times that her awe, and that of others, became normal.

For example, when I was a little over three years old, after my new baby sister was born, my grandfather took our family on our usual Sunday afternoon drive: a delicious ice cream cone was on offer. I was standing in the car, leaning against the back door (no seatbelts back then), admiring the new addition to our family.

As we neared a hairpin turn, I must have leaned against the turn and pulled on the door's handle to balance myself. The door quickly swung open and the air suctioned me out, whisking me away before my parents could even react; the door slammed shut behind me. I flew through the air effortlessly until gravity took hold and I crashed onto the pavement below. I rolled over and over like a bag of trash before stopping completely, exactly in the middle of the hairpin turn.

By that time my father had leapt from the car and was running toward me, not knowing what he would find, all the while fearing someone would round the bend and run over my tiny body. It was now dusk, and as another car closed in on the turn, the driver of that car suddenly pulled off the road and sat there for a moment perplexed, looking toward the hairpin turn where he saw a man running, fear written all over his face. He watched as the man knelt down, turning over whatever was in the road. As he watched, he realized it wasn't a bundle of clothes or a bag of trash, but a young child who had either been hit or had fallen out of the car!

By this time, my grandfather was running toward me also. I was unconscious from the trauma to my head. The driver of the other car joined my family on the roadway as they looked me over. To my father and grandfather's amazement, the driver shared that he had an overwhelming urge to pull off the road and didn't know why until he looked, seeing a child lying directly in his path! The turn was so sharp he wouldn't have seen me in time. He was badly shaken, unnerved, repeating in disbelief, "Dear God, I could have run her over." Needless to say, they were utterly grateful for God's intervention.

My father carried me to the car, where I regained consciousness. Fearing something was broken they raced me to our local doctor's office, where the doctor examined me, but to everyone's amazement nothing was broken—I had just a few cuts and bruises. Still, the doctor wanted me watched closely, fearing a concussion. The following days found me active and playing. At my follow-up appointment, our doctor was still in disbelief, astonished that nothing was wrong. Scratching his head in bewilderment he said, "This is definitely one for the medical books!"

Amazing occurrences seemed to be the norm during my childhood; they were the stories told at family gatherings, remarkable happenings, having no earthly explanation.

At the end of another summer, after a severe asthma attack, I remember calling out to God and Jesus to heal me, my child's prayer of desperation: in my exhausted state, I fell asleep as I stayed in faith. Again, as He had done many times before, Jesus stepped closer and closer to me until I could see him clearly, wanting me to know my suffering was over. This time He communicated that I was to go out onto the beach first thing in the morning.

When I awoke it was as if I had never had an attack. Remembering Jesus's instructions, I told my mother I needed to go to the beach and dressed quickly. My sister Holly wanted to know what all the excitement was about, and I asked her to come along. Taking her hand we headed out together.

The sun shone brightly, the sky a brilliant blue as birds chirped overhead, delighted with another new day. I could see the water ahead of me: the whitecaps glistened as they kissed the shore. It was a glorious day at the water's edge; the tide was high but turning. The beach came into full view as I wondered what Jesus had in store for me.

We took off our sandals and buried our feet in the warm sand. I marveled at the beauty that surrounded us, while thanking Jesus for the day and my healing. Holly played in the sand behind me while I watched the tide recede slowly out to sea. Farther and farther it went, leaving the wet sand behind. Then I began to see what I thought were flat stones scattered thickly over the sandy floor.

My sister distracted me, saying she was tired of waiting. I turned around, explaining there was a surprise for us that she wouldn't want to miss. When I returned my gaze to the beach, I realized that what I had thought were stones were actually hundreds and hundreds of clams, laid out all over the sand. I couldn't believe my eyes!

How I loved clams: steamed clams dipped in melted butter were an all-time favorite of mine. My mother wasn't a seafood lover, so clams were not served often in our home, but any time my mother was willing to cook them I enjoyed a delicious treat. Grabbing my sister's hand, we ran home for a bucket. Soon enough we had filled three buckets' worth, and my mother came out and said it was time to stop!

Our next-door neighbor, who owned a seafood business, called out, "Where are they getting all those clams?" My mother explained that they were just lying atop the beach. Our neighbor went to look for himself and then summoned his men to begin gathering them up. He said, "The clams are so plentiful, my crew won't need to dig today!"

My mother asked if he'd seen anything like it before. He was an elderly gentleman and had sold seafood for most of his life. He answered, "Never in all my years have I seen anything like this. It can only be described as a phenomenon!"

As I washed the clams in preparation for a delicious meal, I thought of how good Jesus was to me; He was the one I turned to when trouble came my way. Enjoying our bounty, I thanked Him for His wonderful surprise and goodness.

But it was during my tenth summer, after experiencing one asthma attack after another, that the most miraculous event occurred, one none of us would ever forget. After gasping for air and praying for help, I went to God as my mother always coaxed me to do and drifted off to sleep. The following morning, like so many others, I was well and healthy again and eager to enjoy a new day.

As I frolicked in the back yard, I spied a beautiful bluebird in one of the trees that bordered our property. He was such a standout amongst the green leaves, hopping along the branches, seeming to be eyeing me as I played in the warm sunshine. Looking up at him, I said, "Hello, boy, you're such a pretty boy, aren't you?"

He sang out as if to answer me, jumping lower and lower on the branches as if he understood what I was saying, head bobbing back and forth, taking in my words. I kept talking and drew closer to the tree he was in. Seeing that he was so at ease with my presence, I stretched out my hand and said, "Come on, boy, I want to see you up close."

He bobbed his head one last time just before taking flight. I watched as he swooped through the air with ease, enthralled as he glided down toward me, surprising me as he landed right in the middle of my palm. Amazingly, we had no fear of each other. He was a gift, I thought, yes, a gift of nature that when beckoned to came unafraid, doing the unthinkable of a wild bird, landing in the palm of my hand! I continued talking to him as he hopped around on my outstretched hand, taking in all my compliments. Up close he was even more magnificent than I had first observed.

Our next-door neighbor's windows provided a full view of our yard. I heard the neighbor call out to my mother, who was working in our kitchen with the window open. My mother came out quickly, fearing something had happened to me, and her sudden movement startled my feathered friend, who flew back to the safety of the tall trees.

Our neighbor joined my mother on our back deck, sharing with her what he'd witnessed. My mother then asked me what happened. I told her about the bluebird, calling him my new friend. She, along with the neighbor, asked me to go back into the yard and call the bird once again, certain his visit was a one-time occurrence.

I went back to the same spot and there he was, so sweet up in the tree, looking down at me as if he knew all I was saying, calling for him once again, "Come on, boy, don't be afraid." Again he took flight, landing perfectly in the middle of my hand.

My mother and the neighbor were shocked. "Maybe he's tame," they suggested, but as soon as they approached me in the yard, the bluebird flew away.

The experience frightened my mother. I was her child who could become desperately ill at any moment and then recover using my faith. Now her child with this great faith was calling a wild bluebird to come to her, and miraculously, without trepidation, the bird did as she asked! In her fear my mother told me to come in for the day, explaining a storm was on its way.

I thought about the picture of Jesus I had seen in my books with the bluebirds all around Him, feeling this bird was God's way of telling me He loved me. I shared this with my mother and wanted to go back outside, but she stood firm, saying the rain would be here soon. The skies did darken, and as the rain pelted down on our roof, I fretted about my new friend. Was he still waiting for me? Had he found shelter? My questions were endless, and looking out every window, I was concerned he was shivering and wet, but I never saw him again.

The rain brought with it a heavy dampness, an irritant to my asthmatic lungs, which began to flare up again. That evening while my father worked late, the attack hit me hard. As I struggled for every ounce of oxygen, my mother moved me to her bedroom where she could watch over me. The tall trees were on that side of the house.

The window shade was up and I looked out at the end of the day, wishing I could see my sweet friend Mr. Bluebird one last time, hoping he'd survive the storm that raged on. All the while my chest was heaving from the damp air and I wanted to cry out but had not enough air to do so. I could barely manage a whisper but said I was so worried about the little bird. Then I prayed for God to heal me once again.

I thought I heard a tapping noise at the windowpane, but I had no energy to sit up and look. My mother went to the window to check. I couldn't hear exactly what she said but I heard her close the blind abruptly. I was too overwhelmed to speak; exhausted, I fell asleep, waking the next morning when I was well again.

Over time I continued to look for my little friend, thinking it odd he never came back to see me…or had he?

Many years later, married with children of my own, we took our annual summer vacation to Massachusetts to visit my family. Unfortunately, our middle child, Blake, suffered from a familiar malady . . . asthma! The damp air was a trigger for him also. On this trip Blake's breathing became labored. To relax him so he could work with the new medication of the time, I told stories of my childhood. He especially loved the spiritual ones.

I told him of the sweet little bluebird, watching over me as I played, when I was just about his age. My story fascinated him and he wanted to hear more. But there was nothing left for me to say—I told him I never saw the little bird again!

My mother, who was sitting on the other side of my son's bed, spoke up, adding sheepishly, "I saw the little bird again but I never told you." This was a revelation to me and I asked her to continue.

She recalled the storm that night with its heavy rains. She said to my son, "Although your mother was barely able to catch her breath, she used all her strength, saying she was worried about the small bird that was out in the storm. I assured her he had found a safe place to stay until the squall was over. As your mother lay there on my bed whispering to God for help, I watched helplessly. And then I heard tapping on the windowpane. I got up to check, thinking the rain had turned to hail. But there was no hail; instead I found the little bluebird, pecking frantically on the windowpane."

My mother admitted that she was shaken. In the middle of that terrible storm, the little bird had found his way to the window in just the bedroom she'd moved me to. "The poor little thing was soaking wet, but he was determined to let me know he was there, even to come in if I'd opened the window slightly." Instead, she said she shooed him away with a toss of her hand and closed the blind.

I asked why she hadn't told me about this years earlier?

She answered, "I know it sounds silly now, but the whole experience terrified me." She explained she was afraid she might lose me and was worried the little bird was a sign that God would take me to my heavenly home.

Thinking of the enormity of my mother's story, I realized the bluebird was God's messenger that summer's eve, a message of hope to one who lay so ill. I knew as a young child all that God could do. In those breathless nights when I believed I'd be healed, He sent sweet gifts, proving our connection. As a child, my asthma attacks were huge mountains I came up against. Yet every time I crossed those mountains, my belief— the intensity of my faith—increased.

I had no idea then about the "life or death" storm I'd face in mid-life, but God knew. My childhood affliction brought me deep into abiding faith, preparing me for my Divine destiny.

As I matured I was blessed with other wonderful opportunities to grow my faith. As a young teenager, for example, my close friend, Tish, and I attended the Billy Graham Crusades at the Boston Gardens, where we would make our way from one of the highest points in the arena, down to and in front of Reverend Graham. The choir sang softly "Oh Lamb of God I Come" as we recommitted our lives to Jesus once again.

With faith firmly established, I grew into young adulthood knowing that whatever obstacles found their way onto my path, love, warmth, family, and most importantly my faith and trust in God would overcome them.

As a young woman I relied on my faith to help soften the agony of losing my grandmother. At her deathbed I whispered in her ear, "Go toward the light, Nan. Remember, when it's my turn, we'll meet at the river." I patted her arm, turned to go, and looked back at her one last time, wondering how I'd ever be able to live without her on this Earth. But as always, God encircled me with His peace and loving care.

Happier times included my precious dating years with George, and then our beautiful wedding and the sweetness of our love for one another. George, then a lieutenant in the U.S. Marine Corps, was sent to Viet Nam, far from home and me. But again I placed my full reliance on God to protect him and to bring him home safely. After a year in harm's way George returned without a scratch. The years passed by as our precious family grew to include two little boys, Merritt and Blake. Soon after, I learned I was pregnant again. I was thrilled until we received orders to go to the Philippine Islands. The thought of uprooting my family and moving halfway around the globe for three years didn't appeal to me. But as I paced the boarding area at the airport, still unsettled about leaving, it was God who gave me the nudge to go along. I prayed, "Heavenly Father, what should I do?" The answer came through my grandfather, who had recently passed away. His voice assured me that I was to go on this journey, giving me peace, as I walked firmly back toward George with complete confidence in my decision.

Amazingly enough, after trusting God, the Philippine Islands turned out to be our best assignment yet. The friendships made there have lasted a lifetime. Shortly after arriving we found two Filipina women, Mina and Garda, to help us with our family. They were our angels planned in the long ago, seeing us safely through our tour of duty and who remain dear to our hearts to this very day. Before leaving, we were even able to assist Mina with her big dream of moving to Canada, where she has lived for decades now, close enough to visit us for many Davis family celebrations over the years.

Our sweet daughter Joanna was born in the Philippines, although her birth was a difficult one. To make matters worse, there was no OB/GYN on the base that night. The relentless labor pains pounded on and on, until I thought I'd lose my ability to continue and possibly lose her. As another exhausting contraction ended I called out to God in desperation, "Oh, Dear Heavenly Father, please help me in this my hour of need. Please take me through this time of terror. Keep me and my baby safe and healthy." Then, suddenly, things changed in that small delivery room. My baby girl came into the world perfectly well and healthy. The pain evaporated as happiness and gratitude took its place.

And of course, throughout my life, there was my dad, who set the bar high with his powerful faith, a shining example for all to see. He was diagnosed with lymphoma at age forty-nine and given only months to live. By God's grace, he lived healthfully for ten more years, living life to the fullest! He beat the odds and was nicknamed by some "The Miracle Man of Massachusetts General Hospital." Finally, on his dying day, with his head hung low and his body failing him, we asked how he had persevered. Mustering his remaining strength, he lifted his head and said, "All you have to do is have faith," summing up his life with that one perfect phrase that has echoed in my mind ever since!

Meditation on the Gaining of Faith

That your faith should not stand in the wisdom of men,
but in the power of God.
1 Corinthians 2:5

So much has been written and spoken about faith over the centuries that I'm certain I cannot add any revelations to the wisdom that is already available. I don't pretend to have a fail-safe formula for you to follow if you desire to build and sustain your faith in God—it is a deeply personal journey that can only occur after we as individuals have let go of all distractions from faith and all rationales about why we shouldn't bother to grow our faith.

I do know one thing with complete and unalterable certainty, however: once we give ourselves over to desiring faith, our lives change forever, and they change in the greatest and most satisfying ways. Here are some simple techniques for starting to think about faith, beginning with the world around us:

Allow your senses to recognize that the essence of God is everywhere, from a newborn baby to a flower pushing its way through the earth and blossoming. God's handiwork is omnipresent and His existence speaks to us daily in every direction we turn. He provides us with endless beauty to help focus our awareness on His goodness, if only we look and listen.

Accept the fact that faith is about establishing a relationship with an entity we cannot actually see or touch—obviously a difficult concept for human beings who live in a rational, tactile world. But faith can only take root and grow if we prepare an accepting piece of ground for it, a well-tilled and nourished soul, not a rational, nit-picking mind.

Be in action for God to be in action. Sitting by passively and hoping that faith will one day come to us is not a plan. We must work in concert with God to develop our personal, unique faith in Him, using the means and tools He gives us.

For example, we can grow our faith by memorizing Bible passages that speak to us deeply, and then meditate on these passages daily. We can fill our minds with positive stories and thoughts, avoiding the cynicism that the world is all too anxious to bestow on us. We can communicate with God throughout the day, thanking Him for all He has done, being grateful in all things no matter how small or routine. We can strive to be the best person we can possibly be as an example of His love.

Any relationship, by definition, is a two-way street, and our relationship with God is no different. We must do our part, through prayer, devotion, and action, to walk more closely with Him. He is always calling and whispering our name, wanting us to awaken spiritually and be in touch with Him through prayer and trust. When we lower the volume of our daily lives and listen intently for God's whisper, the whisper begins to fill our lives with passionate intensity. When we simply believe, we see with perfect clarity the miracles He performs daily, all around us, in every atom of the space in which we live.

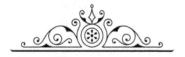

Section II
The Gift of Adversity

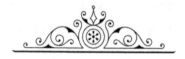

Prelude

When you face adversity, you need to remind yourself that whatever is trying to defeat you could very well be what God will use to promote you.
Joel Osteen

By the early 1980s, I was a successful businesswoman with a strong background in finance. I was offered a new opportunity at a Professional Corporation in northern Virginia as Director of Business Development, my title encompassing never-ending responsibilities. Yet, I happily put in long hours and enjoyed the daily challenge of growing the company. Finding buildings and negotiating their purchase or lease became my specialty, expanding our availability to our clients. The work required intense energy, concentration, and creativity, but in the beginning I didn't view these requirements as stressful—just the opposite, in fact; I thrived on the challenge.

Early on I had hired an assistant, Katy, a standout, bubbly personality with strong sales ability. She and I formed an unbeatable team on both professional and personal levels, and her support proved crucial to my wellbeing in the years ahead. It's also where I first met Ben, one of the professionals who worked two days a week for the corporation, having a small business of his own. He admired my business acumen, looking to me for new ideas and tips on how to grow his own company. We complemented each other in many ways, sharing the added bonus of being good friends.

After several years of working there I had made a name for myself and decided to leave the corporation and all its pressure; Katy gave her notice, too. A month later Ben contacted me, deciding it was time to expand his company, and approached me to help him do just that. He wanted to hire Katy as well, so we sealed the deal and set off on an exciting new venture.

Through more hard work and tireless dedication our business became a model for success. My job was secure and I had excellent income and benefits. I was confident that the people who worked at the business served our clients with the utmost professionalism.

Before long our small city office could no longer support the growth we experienced: my quest began to find a larger building to meet our needs. My search along with negotiations took two years. Several times during that time frame, just when I thought everything was set, things fell apart for one reason or another. There would be no contract, no new building, and no move, forcing me to start the search anew. This pursuit was done simultaneously while running businesses at several locations. However, one day my hard work paid off, and I found the perfect place, a building near a main thoroughfare, near many of our clientele.

Motivated by the find, I negotiated an incredible twenty-year lease, ensuring Ben's company time and room to grow. Contracts were signed, furnishings purchased; a move-in date lay ahead.

On my drive to work each day, I often prayed, thankful for my many blessings as the beauty of nature touched my spirit. I took pride in my job, grateful for all God helped me to accomplish, inspiring me to be the best I could be for others as well as myself.

But unexpectedly, on a fateful day in the mid-1990s, all the peace and success we enjoyed suddenly changed. We discovered that a trusted employee had embezzled and spent large sums of money, throwing us into chaos. Years' worth of accounting was now suspect and needed to be scrutinized and unraveled. We called outside firms to possibly resolve the problem, but their costs were prohibitive. Even if they could have solved the puzzle with all its missing pieces, we were advised that we would still need face-to-face resolution with each client, a formidable, time-consuming, and embarrassing prospect.

The embezzler was convicted and sent to jail, a small consolation to me as I struggled mightily to keep the business afloat. I didn't realize it then, but looking back now, the day the jail cell closed on our former employee was the day I was incarcerated, too! As the person in charge of the company's business, the pressure fell heaviest on me to resolve the multitude of accounts before we could bill again. I had to put together a team of employees to begin the daunting task, adding more work to our already encumbered days.

We had taken the usual loans to outfit the new building, but now we needed a large loan to tide us over while we resolved falsified accounts we couldn't collect on. This unforeseen and unfortunate set of circumstances weighed heavily on the overall future and ultimately the financial success of the company. We needed help and we needed it now.

The stress of holding the business together as creditors expected their due and the horrible distraction from our normal, forward-looking development plans began taking their toll on me. My professional life was transformed from energizing and fulfilling to a daily grind of all-consuming stress. Joy drained out of me as resolution of the problem dragged on for several years, sapping my energy and focus despite my intense efforts to hold everything together.

This professional stress became interwoven with health concerns that I should have taken seriously. One day, out of the blue, I developed an agonizing pain in my neck that prevented me from turning my head. Katy was frightened and rushed me to the doctor, who diagnosed severe muscle lock-up, caused by stress. After several weeks of physical therapy the pain abated, but not before the doctor apprised me of what was happening. He explained that stress had gone too far when it moved from my mind to my body, causing physical damage. He warned me, "Unless you make changes in your professional life, your stress will continue to manifest itself in physical and unpredictable ways."

It was a frightening statement, yet I dismissed it! I wanted to believe that I was healthy and strong and nothing could happen to me. Too many people depended on my dedication to the business, on my total commitment to making things right. I wouldn't give up, continuing to push myself relentlessly, more concerned about saving a company than attending to my own health.

In the fall of 1997, as the stress continued to build, I felt a sharp pain in the left side of my abdomen. I suspected an ovarian cyst, based on an experience I had had years before, but I tried to ignore this new and excruciating pain, hoping it would go away. There was always so much more to do for the company!

Eventually, though, the pain became so severe that I was forced to see my gynecologist, who ordered an abdominal sonogram as well as my yearly mammogram. During the exam, I mentioned that the fibroids in my left breast had been bothering me, but the doctor said he didn't feel anything unusual.

Returning for the follow-up appointment, my gynecologist said the sonogram revealed a small ovarian cyst, as I had suspected, and my mammogram was normal. He recommended the birth control pill as standard treatment for the cyst, adding I might notice a harmless change in my breast tissue due to increased estrogen levels caused by the pill. He assured me it would be nothing to worry about. I agreed to the treatment. I was tired of the pain and ready to try anything at that point.

My doctor then guided my right hand to the fibrous area in my left breast, wanting me to be familiar with the fibroid shelf there and showing me how to recognize any changes through self-examination.

Those few simple moments of instruction proved to be another gift from God, as the months ahead would soon reveal.

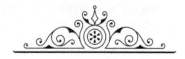

Shadows

Hear my cry, O God; attend unto my prayer. From the end
of the earth will I cry unto thee, when my heart is overwhelmed:
lead me to the rock that is higher than I.
Psalm 61:1–2 (KJV)

On November 30, 1997, I was preparing for a romantic evening with my husband to celebrate our wedding anniversary. Each year we take turns planning our special day; this year it was George's turn and I was excited to see what surprises he had in store. He had hinted that it would be a dressy evening, so I had purchased just the right dress to wow him.

After showering I proceeded to my dressing room, where I could depend on the mirrors and bright lights to point out any flaws on my body. I took off the wet towel and glanced at my reflection, thinking not too bad for almost forty-nine years old! I was a walker, priding myself on taking good care of my figure. As I patted myself dry from the neck down, I reached my full breasts, inherited from my mother and grandmother. I smiled, thinking of the pretty black bra and panties that lay on my bed, buying them especially for tonight.

Then something in the mirror caught my eye and momentarily took my breath away: I thought I saw a light gray shadow above my left nipple. I turned the lights up brighter and looked from every angle, but the shadow seemed to disappear. Had I imagined it?

Just then George came through our bedroom door with all sorts of gifts in his hands and a big smile on his face, finding me undressed. But I was alarmed, which he quickly saw written all over my face.

"What's wrong, honey?"

"I thought I saw some shading above my left nipple. Can you take a closer look?"

Playfully he teased, "Okay, I'm the doctor, now let me examine your breast."

"Stop fooling around. This is scaring me to death!"

Then he got serious, studying my nipple area, and finally said, "Nope... no shading, just those same beautiful breasts I've been looking at for twenty-eight years now."

He hugged me tight. "I know you've been under a lot of stress and your ovary's been bothering you, but you're fine. Stop worrying about yourself and get ready so we can enjoy our evening." He winked at me, leaving the room to take his shower.

Taking one last look in the mirror, I convinced myself I had imagined the shadow. Maybe next year I'd stop concentrating so much on the company's problems and take better care of myself, knowing I needed to. But for tonight, anyway, I was determined to put it all to rest and enjoy my anniversary.

George did not disappoint on the arrangements. We had a wonderful evening at one of our favorite places, a beautiful rooftop restaurant overlooking the Potomac River and the lights of our nation's capital. We held hands and gazed at one another, enjoying our celebratory evening alone, lost in our own world.

At work the next day as I wrote December on my correspondence, I could hardly believe another year was coming to an end.

Just before our annual Christmas party I called a meeting, once again telling Ben I couldn't continue to juggle the unresolved financial issues. The burden was affecting my health and he needed to find an answer immediately. I reminded him that we had discussed the possibility that he might ask a well-off uncle of his for a loan. Once again he assured Katy and me that he'd think it over. I understood that he might be reluctant to ask a relative for money, but I knew instinctively that this particular relative, a kind, generous-spirited older man, would be happy to help. It was frustrating that Ben would not approach him. The company desperately needed his assistance.

As Katy and I drove to the Christmas party together, she confided she was drained from all the burdens and pressures of the past few years.

"I wish I could leave and start over in a new job that was just a job!" she exclaimed.

I never thought I'd hear myself say it aloud, but I answered, "I want out, too!"

Katy swiveled her head in surprise.

"I'm drained! I am simply worn out!" I continued. But I quickly reminded her that leaving Ben would mean we'd no longer work together.

"No matter how crazy things have been in these past years, Katy, we've always had each other to lean on. I can't imagine not seeing you every day."

She turned away and lowered her voice. "I never thought about that," she replied sadly.

Now Katy begged, "Cath, what about your dream, can't you make it happen so we can be rid of this rat race?"

She was referring to a recurring dream I had shared with her over the years. I'm not normally a person who remembers dreams, but every so often one stands out. The dream always began with me standing in the wings of a large auditorium. After hearing my introduction I walked to the podium as women clapped enthusiastically, and I saw Katy in the audience distributing a book that instinctively I knew I'd written. As she made her way to the far wall, I turned to introduce her. In my dream Katy would throw me a kiss; in turn I'd throw one back. At this juncture the dream always ended. When I awoke, I remembered the feeling of joy I experienced on that stage.

Katy loved to analyze and probe. "But where were we, Cath, and what were we doing?"

The truth is, I wasn't sure. It did seem odd, though, that year after year the dream repeated itself.

Now Katy said, "Maybe it's a sign, Cath? You always have great ideas. Maybe you could start a consulting company and I'll go to work for you and we'll travel together."

I answered, "Even if I could make it happen, what about Ben? After all, he depends on us. We couldn't just walk out the door now for our own self-gain. What would happen to the company?"

Katy was highly conscientious, too, and I knew my words would work on her heart. We rode in silence for a few minutes, our conversation lingering in the air. As we arrived at the party I asked her what she thought.

She sighed. "I guess you're right, Cath, we'll have to see it through."

We were trapped for now, believing there was no way out. Together we made a new commitment to Ben and his company for the New Year of 1998. During the party I watched Ben enjoy himself. For that matter we were all enjoying ourselves. I just knew he finally understood: he would take action to solve our problems immediately. Next year would be a great New Year for us in the business. Our difficulties would be resolved with a loan from his uncle, getting us back on track, allowing us to concentrate on growing the business once again. Just thinking about it put a smile on my face.

I was lost in my thoughts until the surrounding chatter and festivity subsided. That's when reality set in, and I knew I was fooling myself.

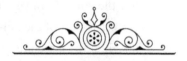

The River of Denial

Come to me, all you who are weary and burdened, and I
will give you rest. Take my yoke upon you and learn from me,
for I am gentle and humble in heart, and you will find rest for
your souls. For my yoke is easy and my burden is light.
Matthew 11: 28–31

Our holidays at home that year were filled with the warmth and togetherness our family cherishes. Our boys were home from college, filling the house with their energy. When they weren't playing with our two big dogs—a Rottweiler named Hildy and an Akita named Kuma—or visiting friends, they spent much of their time trying to coax their sister, Joanna, to be the third Davis to attend Marshall University in the fall. She was having none of it, wanting to be away from their watchful eyes. We celebrated the season with parties and much cheer.

But while enjoying each day of the season, my mind continued to obsess about the shaded area I thought I had seen above my nipple weeks earlier. I tried to calm myself by reviewing all the reasons I was healthy: I walked on the treadmill every day, ate right, and kept my weight under control. Then I thought about the stress from my job. I had no good answer to that nagging issue. I steered clear of the full-length mirror after showering, not wanting to "imagine" the discolored area again. After all, I assured myself, I'd just seen my gynecologist in November.

Before I could blink, or so it seemed, we were bidding farewell to the boys as their Christmas vacation came to an end. I headed back to work, where normally I looked forward to the New Year. Goals were set, plans were made, hard work would solve all problems, or so I always believed, but this time things were different. Once back at my desk I busily scheduled meetings, assessed my to do list, and tackled a mile-high pile of projects, all of which kept me away from the burning question: had Ben spoken to his uncle about a loan?

He and I met for lunch several times in the first few weeks of January, but with so many other issues to discuss, I hadn't asked him about the loan request. Maybe I didn't want to hear his answer. But the stress and strain mounted with each new week. The joy I had felt during the holidays quickly receded to distant memory as I continued to work long hours. But I also knew with growing certainty that something needed to change.

One afternoon, depleted of energy, I decided to leave work at the normal time, unheard of for me. Once home I turned on the TV to catch the Oprah Winfrey show, a luxury to me. This day her guest was Sarah Ban Breathnach, author of *Simple Abundance*, talking about simplicity and gratefulness for simple things. Sarah's words filled me up— my soul longed for a simpler life. The next day I purchased her book, hoping it would help me regain some balance and understand my real purpose in this life. I prayed to God for His intervention and to see me through the demanding time ahead. I asked God to bring back the joy in my life, telling Him I couldn't continue to deal with all the stress and pressure much longer.

During the daily phone call my sister Holly and I share, I told her about *Simple Abundance* and admitted my desperation for change. I also finally confessed my worry about seeing the faint grayish shadow above my nipple in November. She was instantly concerned and urged an immediate visit to the doctor. As usual, though, my reflexive answer was filled with excuses: I was too busy at work; the doctor had just seen me two months earlier, and so on. I continued with my excuses but she insisted, "Cath, it's your life we're talking about here," making me promise to schedule a follow-up appointment. Why do we need others to push us so hard to take care of ourselves, I wondered?

By the end of January Ben had yet to mention anything about the loan. I had resolved to confront him at our next business luncheon. He entered the restaurant as if he hadn't a care in the world. We reviewed important issues pertinent to the company, marking them off in my notebook one by one. Then we sat back and went to the personal side of our lives. He asked about my children, I asked about his; we were good friends, enjoying each other's company. Then I asked, "Did you speak with your uncle during the holidays about a loan?"

He looked guilt-stricken, saying that he hadn't. He said he just felt so confident that I would make everything right for the company—we wouldn't need the outside money.

I felt sick. This was the body blow I had feared was coming.

On our way back to the office, Ben drove behind me. I could see him in my rear view mirror, peaceful and relaxed, and I realized he was never going to speak to his uncle or anyone else for that matter. In that moment the load I carried was so heavy I could barely catch my breath. I had already suffered several health warnings but now my spirit was dying.

Later that day, while driving home, my left nipple was itchy again as it had been on and off all month. This time the nipple area seemed hard to the touch, its texture different, but as usual I told myself I was fine. As I turned down our street, home never looked so welcoming, with my family and a hot meal waiting inside.

Pulling in the driveway I decided not to tell George about my meeting with Ben, knowing that he'd urge me to look for another job immediately. I knew as I turned the doorknob there was nothing more I could do tonight anyway. I walked through the door, relishing the aroma of a crockpot full of home-cooked food. George and Joanna were putting the meal on the table as I walked in the kitchen. I gave each a hug and kiss as we sat down to catch up with each other's day.

After the respite of dinner I stood at the kitchen sink, lost in thought, washing out the crockpot. I dwelled on what would happen to the business. Joanna came to say goodnight. George called out he was taking the dogs for their final outing.

I went to my room to take a fast shower, getting in and out quickly. As I dried myself in front of the mirror I tried to keep my eyes averted, fearing what I might see on my left breast, but I couldn't help it, I looked anyway. At a glance all seemed fine. Still, I remembered the breast's odd texture on the way home. Wanting to put my incessant worrying to rest, I decided to lie on the bed for self-examination as my doctor had shown me.

First, my fingertips explored my right breast: all seemed normal. Moving to my left breast, its texture was definitely different. I pushed down, noting the outline of the fibroid shelf. Pressing deeper, my fingers suddenly bumped into something, definitely something I had never felt before. My heart skipped a very large beat. Just then George came into our bedroom.

"Honey, what are you doing?"

"Something feels odd in my left breast. It's constantly itchy, so I wanted to do a self-exam."

"OK, but remember, your gynecologist said there could be changes in your fibroid shelf."

Taking George's hand, I pulled him down on the bed beside me and guided his fingertips to the spot in question. He felt the area and I watched his face for expression but saw no alarm.

"Honey, it's your fibroid shelf or a change from the pill, but it's nothing for you to worry about."

They were just the words I wanted to hear. We readied ourselves for bed and I snuggled into his arms for the night.

Now That's a Boston Girl for You

The Lord is my light and my salvation; whom shall I fear? The Lord is the strength of my life; of whom shall I be afraid?
Psalm 27:1

*D*espite a good night's sleep, my new finding troubled me, and I wondered in the morning if I should stop taking the pill, although I didn't want to return to the severe abdominal pain I had been experiencing. Just then my mother called, and I told her about the changes in my fibroid shelf. She thought she recalled my great aunt having similar problems, possibly having the fibroids surgically removed. Now that seemed like something worth discussing with my doctor at a new appointment.

After I arrived at work, Katy followed me into my office for a brief morning meeting, pouring me a cup of freshly brewed coffee. After we discussed the business of the day, I told her I was calling my doctor about the enlargement of my fibroid. With my office door closed I came around my desk and stood before Katy, asking her to feel through my sweater the hardness above my nipple area. Taking her hand I guided her fingertips. I could see her shock as she pulled back.

"Cath, that doesn't feel normal. You need to call your doctor *right away.*"

After months of making excuses, after weeks of rationalizing my fear, I finally picked up the phone and made the call. After a quick discussion with the doctor's coordinator, she told me to come in first thing the next day. I alerted Ben about the appointment, sharing with him the problem I was experiencing and adding that the constant stress from work was killing me!

The next morning my doctor came through the door, chatting casually. I told him my ovarian pain was gone but now my fibroid was enlarged. As he began the exam I watched his face as his fingertips touched the growing area in my left breast. He went back and forth several times, probing gently, looking off into space. Although he was calm I could easily see he was troubled. Finally, he looked at me and said, "It's a mass of some sort, possibly a water-filled cyst."

He reviewed my chart, noting the mass wasn't there in June when I had my last mammogram. Without further ado he said he was sending me to radiology as soon as possible today for a sonogram and another mammogram. He said to remain in the radiologist's office after the tests were done and he would call me on the phone in the waiting room with further instructions.

Everything was happening so fast and my mind was racing. I said to him, "You're not concerned about this, are you? Or should I say it's nothing I should be concerned about, is it?"

He replied, "It could simply be a water-filled cyst, Cathy, and if that's the case I'll have you come back to the office today and I'll drain it."

Radiology could see me at 2:30, and I left his office with appointment in hand, knowing this was nothing serious.

On that cold and rainy day in February I drove to my office, still trying to digest what had happened that morning. Pulling the hood of my coat over my head, I made a mad dash for the front door. Katy called from the city office to see how everything had gone. A cyst didn't sound threatening to either of us, so we continued to talk about issues pertinent to the company.

The rain wasn't letting up but it was time to meet George for lunch. We went to a nearby Chinese restaurant for soup and hot tea, the perfect remedy for a cold and wet day. I told him what the doctor found and he insisted on going with me to radiology. I asked him if he was worried. Reaching for my hand across the table he said, "No, honey, I'm sure it's nothing. I just want to be there for you."

We finished our lunch and made our way across town to the radiologist's office. Since I was being worked into the schedule, I knew a wait was ahead of us. After we sat down, George read over some work he had brought with him. I began talking to God, as I often do in situations I have no control over, giving the problem to Him as I waited. When they called my name, George smiled up at me as I left.

They took the mammogram first, after which I was asked to wait in the changing room while films were developed. The radiologist did not ask for further x-rays, which I took as a good sign. I moved right along to the sonogram: all was going well. The technician was a pleasant young woman who spoke calmly and remained upbeat as she worked. I looked for any sign of unease, yet I saw none. When she finished I returned to the waiting room and sat down next to George with a smile on my face.

"How did it go, honey?"

"Great, there were no retakes and no one seemed alarmed by what they saw."

George leaned over and kissed me on the cheek. "I know that made you feel better. I told you it would be fine."

Just then the nurse asked me to pick up the wall phone to speak with my gynecologist. In all the years of coming in for mammograms, I had never noticed the wall phone before, and neither could I have imagined what it was used for. Now my gynecologist was telling me to come directly back to his office and to bring the sonogram with me, although he didn't seem alarmed. I collected the sonogram and we drove back to his building.

When we arrived I signed in and left the sonogram with the receptionist. Soon after that we were ushered into my doctor's private office. He walked in with his referral pad in hand. He held the sonogram over our heads to the light in the ceiling and said, "See the object shaped like a large goose egg? Well, that's what's lying under your fibroid shelf."

I asked, "Is it a water-filled cyst?"

"The radiologist doesn't believe so."

My heart began to race. "What is it then?"

"That's just it, we don't know right now. That's why I'm giving you this referral. The mass needs to be biopsied."

The word biopsy didn't sound like a good word to me. I stood next to my doctor and said, "We're not talking about cancer, are we?" Again he held the picture above our heads and we stared at what looked exactly like a big goose egg.

"The radiologist said it's large but it has no tentacles, so whatever it is we've hopefully caught it early."

I pressed on, "What do you think it could be?"

He studied the picture for another few seconds and said, "You've had normal mammograms every year. It could be a benign tumor that's grown under your shelf, but whatever it is I want it removed. My staff is getting you an appointment with the surgeon as we speak. You'll enjoy him—he was schooled up north."

We set up the appointment with the surgeon for Thursday morning. George and I put on our warm coats to face the cold, drizzly weather that awaited us. He walked me to my car, kissing me before I got in and saying, "Honey, it's going to be fine, don't let your mind run wild on your ride home. You're a healthy woman and you know it."

I did know it, and smiling I patted his cheek.

Thursday morning George and I met with the surgeon, who entered the room with my sonogram and doctors' reports with him. We shook hands and I asked what he thought of the sonogram. He said he'd need to perform the needle biopsy to better understand what was going on. As he examined my left breast he explained how the biopsy was performed. The procedure didn't sound overly distressing.

I told him I heard he was schooled up north. He noted my accent and asked where I was from. When I replied Duxbury on the South Shore he said he knew of the area. Then he asked if I'd need some numbing cream before performing the biopsy. I answered, "No, I think I'll be fine." He looked at his nurse and said, "Now that's a Boston girl for you. They make 'em tough up there!"

That broke the ice and we all laughed. A definite rapport was building quickly between this surgeon and me. He relaxed and so did I. He then began the biopsy by inserting a long needle into the area of concern. He pulled the syringe out and asked me to sit up as he looked closely at the sample he'd collected.

Then he said, "I must tell you when I first viewed your sonogram and read the radiologist's report, I was concerned."

I thought to myself, "concerned about what?" My heart began to pound and I wondered, "Is he talking about cancer?"

He continued, "But now that I've seen your biopsy with my own eyes, and it's filled with fluid, I'm relieved. Of course I'll send the biopsy to the lab for official results, which will come back as either benign, inconclusive, or conclusive, meaning cancerous."

"What do you think my result will be?"

"I feel confident they will be either benign or inconclusive. Don't worry if it comes back inconclusive. That just means I didn't get enough tissue sample on the first try." Summing up his assessment he said, "I think you have a benign tumor growing under your fibroid shelf. But since I never leave anything growing in the breast, we need to schedule surgery."

"So I have nothing to be concerned about?"

He smiled and said, "That's right."

He then instructed me to call his office the following Thursday to speak with a phone nurse, who would give me my biopsy results. I also needed to meet with his attending nurse to set up a surgical date. While dressing, I thanked God for this easy answer. I had been certain it wasn't anything serious, but it was still good to hear the surgeon say I had nothing to worry about.

I followed the nurse to a room where surgeries were scheduled. Since she had been in the room throughout the procedure, I asked if the surgeon ever told patients not to worry if he suspected something else. She answered strongly, "No, he would never make the statement he made to you unless he was certain of your outcome."

I thanked her, leaving to meet George in the waiting room where he was working on his laptop. I smiled as I walked toward him. He looked up and said, "All set, honey?" I shook my head yes. He gathered his things, put his coat on, and helped me with mine. On the ride back I told him what the surgeon said, adding that I needed to have the growth removed in the near future. He took my hand and said, "I knew it was something simple, honey."

But the thought of surgery was unsettling, since I experience horrendous side effects from anesthesia. Looking straight ahead I said, "I just hate to go through surgery, with the nausea and dizziness that go with it."

George replied, "No one wants you to have surgery, honey, but it's much better than what he could have told you today."

I turned to him, asking if he had suspected cancer?

"I never thought you had cancer. I felt strongly your problem was simple. After all, honey, you've had normal mammograms every year since you were forty. I saw women in the surgeon's office today who really looked sick, so different from you. I'm grateful your problem is so simple." I could see where he was going with this conversation. The growth obviously developed over the past few months due to the estrogen in the birth control pill. My gynecologist ordered a mammogram along with the sonogram to prove the growth's recent development.

George reminded me how blessed we were. We worked hard and kept ourselves healthy, we had a great family, enjoyed a wonderful life-style, and had all the trappings of a successful life together. He was right, what was I whining about? I needed surgery to remove a benign growth, I might even get sick from the anesthesia, but I was definitely more fortunate than the other women in the surgeon's office today!

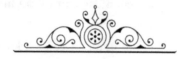

The Day of Reckoning

But he knows the way that I take, when he has tested me,
I will come forth as gold.
Job 23:10

week of waiting for lab results lay ahead of us. I called my family on a conference call, telling them what the surgeon had to say, explaining the three possible results of a biopsy. Holly and my mother made me promise to come to Boston for a second opinion, even if the results were inconclusive. Holly's husband, Robert, was Chief Executive Officer of a cancer research company and had connections with the best doctors in the city. He could get me an appointment with a team of breast specialists quickly.

I reassured them, saying I was certain my results would be benign. I prayed each night for that simple outcome, eliminating a trip to Boston for further testing.

The week passed by quickly, and before I knew it, Thursday, February 12, was upon me. In the beginning of the New Year I had changed the company's hours of operation on Thursdays to open at noon and close in the early evening, so I was still at home when George left for work. He told me to have a good day and to call him as soon as I had spoken with the phone nurse.

As he was leaving the room I said, "George, I know this sounds silly, but what if they tell me something else today?"

"Something else like what?"

"You know, something bad."

He replied, "You're a healthy woman, and you have nothing to be concerned about." He almost sounded bothered by my question, and I felt silly to have asked it out loud.

Soon after, as Joanna was leaving for school, she hugged me goodbye and said, "I know the news will be good today, Mom." I told her I was certain of it. She was a wonderful child, my only daughter, and we were attached at the hip. She reminded me to pick up the balloons for the Mother and Daughter Valentines dinner we had plans for that evening at a local restaurant.

Later that morning I was busy getting ready for work when our housekeeper Anna knocked at the front door. I let her in and we chatted a bit. Throughout the years Anna and I had gone through many difficult times together: the death of her mother, illnesses in her family, and a breast cancer scare. I had prayed for her daily, reminding her God would see her through all difficulties. Thankfully, her biopsy the year before had revealed no cancer!

She asked if I'd talked to my surgeon's office yet, and I told her I was going to call once I was ready for work. She said she'd been praying for me and I thanked her for her kindness. George then called to ask if I had any news yet. I told him I was getting ready to make the call, assuring him that the surgeon's office would have called me first thing in the morning if anything were wrong with my results.

Oddly enough during George's morning meeting, he learned he was being sent to Boston for the next two weeks on business. He asked if I could take some time off and visit him during his two-week stay. Before I could answer, my gynecologist's office beeped in, and I told George I'd call him back later.

It was the office administrator, whom I'd known for years. My doctor asked her to give me a call to see if I'd heard from the surgeon's office yet. I could hear the concern in her voice. I explained that the surgeon felt strongly I had nothing to be concerned about. She seemed puzzled by my comment, but just then I remembered I hadn't received my mammogram report yet and asked if it was in my file.

I could hear her shuffling through my chart when she answered, "Here it is, Cathy, your results were normal." I was confused, to say the least.

"How could the mammogram be normal with a growth the size of a goose egg in my breast?"

I asked her to look again, to check the dates. Was this the mammogram taken the same day as the sonogram? She knew it was a valid question and humored me as she checked the report again.

"I have your report in front of me, written exactly the same day as the sonogram. 'No Suspicious Findings–Normal.'"

Fear gripped my mind and body as I translated this information rapidly. My yearly mammogram, my means of safeguarding myself from any suspicious growths, was still reading normal when a huge growth existed under my fibroid shelf: the mammogram completely missed it! I told her I had to go, I needed to contact the surgeon right away.

Now I knew I hadn't been safe all these years. How long had this growth been developing and what in God's name was it? I closed my bedroom door as I shuffled through my purse to find the surgeon's card. I needed to speak to his phone nurse right away. I sat on the edge of my bed in my suit and high heels, ready to go to work once I got this clarified.

The receptionist greeted me cheerfully, and before connecting me to the phone nurse she explained how busy they were that day. When she came back on the line, she said it might take a few more minutes. I thanked her as she placed me on hold again. The hold was beyond tedious. I prayed as I waited.

When the line opened up again, a man spoke my name in sadness. I knew before he identified himself it was the surgeon. He continued, saying he was very sorry to give me this news over the phone, but the biopsy came back conclusive: it was breast cancer! And it was quite serious, aggressive breast cancer stage III.

My voice quivered as I asked, "How can this be possible? You seemed so certain last week that it was nothing to be concerned about."

He apologized, explaining that after receiving the report this morning, he called the lab himself in disbelief, asking to speak directly to the head pathologist, a friend of his. He told her my biopsy hadn't appeared cancerous in any way. She offered to run the test herself to be certain.

Then he said, "Cathy, I just got off the phone with her, she ran the test a second time herself, she's certain it's aggressive breast cancer and is willing to bet her job on it."

"So what do I do now and what does this mean to me?"

He lowered his voice and replied, "Your cancer is growing by leaps and bounds, and the mass needs to be removed as quickly as possible. We need to schedule a mastectomy immediately."

Then his voice lowered even further and he said, "If I had even remotely suspected this outcome, I would have had you come to my office for the results, never over the phone like this. Again, I'm terribly sorry."

I must have said goodbye but I can't remember. I'd been pacing back and forth like a caged animal, trying to process the terrifying news. Aggressive breast cancer—not regular but aggressive! My mind was whirling from shock.

I dialed George's office; he was in a meeting. I told his secretary it was urgent. George answered moments later, and I was aggravated, remembering what he'd said that morning, reminding me how healthy I was and how silly I'd been to question otherwise.

As he answered the phone I blurted out, "Well, you were right, it isn't breast cancer…instead, it's much worse, it's aggressive breast cancer."

He demanded, "Who gave you this information?" I recapped my conversation with the surgeon. George was irate. Surely they'd made a mistake, and he threatened to sue the lot of them for upsetting me like this. He told me to hang up and sit tight. He was calling the surgeon and the lab right away to get to the bottom of this ridiculous diagnosis.

My next thought was to call Katy, who had been waiting to hear that all was well. She answered with her usual cheerful greeting, but when I went to speak, no words came out. I tried again but still nothing. She could tell someone was on the line and repeated, "Hello, may I help you?" Finally my voice box issued a distressed sound, managing to whisper a pitiful "Katy."

I could hear the panic in Katy's voice as she asked loudly, "Cath, is it you? Oh my God, Cath, what did they say?"

Somehow I cried out "It's breast cancer." Katy screamed and dropped the phone. It bounced several times. I stayed on the line, listening to the commotion. Minutes later another employee picked up the phone and asked sadly, "Cath, is it really breast cancer?"

"Yes," I whispered.

She replied, "I'm sure they've caught it early, right?"

Barely able to repeat the words, I said, "The surgeon says it's aggressive breast cancer."

She gasped in horror. My throat was bone dry but somehow I asked to speak to Katy again. I was told she had gone to tell Ben, and then grabbed her coat and ran out the front door crying. She was probably on her way to my house.

I pushed the off button on the phone and reached to place it back in its cradle: a futile attempt, as my hand shook out of control. Then my entire body began to shake and my teeth chattered. Shock and hysteria took over as I began screaming, trying to get out of my room. I couldn't turn the doorknob, but I needed to escape, far away from that stunning phone call. The result I never thought I'd hear had my name on it!

Somehow I managed to turn the knob. Free at last I ran down the hallway screaming as if someone were chasing me, trying to get to me, trying to kill me. As I turned the corner I crashed into Anna, who was carrying an armful of folded towels. She dropped the laundry and began screaming "Oh my God, no!" We fell into each other's arms, collapsing to our knees and holding on to one another as we sobbed.

My big dogs ran up the stairs, barking and sniffing as they ran round us, trying to protect me from whatever was happening, but they couldn't protect me from this! Anna helped me to the chair by our front window. I saw Katy's car make the turn, and from my bird's eye view I could see she was crying.

Katy's brother, one year younger than she, had suffered a terrible death from cancer only five years earlier. She was at his side for the two years he went through one chemotherapy after another. I knew today all those emotions would be resurrected. She sat there in her car trying to gather strength, having no choice but to go on this journey again, this time as her best friend was forced to fight the insidious disease.

When I opened the door I knew our lives would never be the same. She entered my house with tears still streaming. She hugged me, yet we spoke not a word. Turning, we walked into my kitchen and sat at the table. We laid our foreheads on our arms and wept audibly for half an hour, stopping only for tissues.

All cried out, we regained some composure, and Katy said, pleadingly, "Why you, Cath, you're so good, why you?" I didn't have an answer at the time.

I asked her if she had told Ben. She said yes, she had interrupted him momentarily during a meeting with a client to whisper the news in his ear. He was distraught enough to end the meeting abruptly and retreat to his private office.

At that point Anna interrupted Katy and me to ask if she could leave for the day. She was shaken to the core, and I thanked her for being with me, telling her she could go. She left, saying I'd be in her prayers. Katy said she'd leave as soon as George arrived home, wanting to give us our privacy. Just then we heard the garage door open, signaling his arrival. As George entered the kitchen, Katy shook her head in disbelief, and reached up to give him a hug before departing. I walked her to the front door as she kissed me on the cheek. "Know you'll be in my prayers," she said.

George and I stared at one another. He pulled me close and said, "We'll face this together, honey, just like we've faced everything else that's come our way." I lay my head on his chest. Neither of us spoke a word. There were no words to say. We just stood in the middle of our kitchen and comforted each other.

Later on, we talked, deciding not to tell our boys about this diagnosis over the phone. They were coming home for the weekend to celebrate one of our family's favorite holidays, Valentine's Day, and also to celebrate Joanna's acceptance at Marshall University. She had finally given in to their coaxing!

We planned to tell Joanna when she arrived home from school. In the meantime I knew I needed to tell my mother and sisters. George encouraged me to get it over with; time wouldn't make the calls any easier.

I dialed my mother's number first, praying she wouldn't be home so I could just leave a simple message. I sighed with relief when her answering machine came on. "Mom, the news today wasn't good. When you call back please be strong as I'll need your strength during this difficult time."

I could just imagine my mother coming in from work, humming one of her favorite tunes. In her happy state she'd go straight to her answering machine, expecting the message that all was well. Hearing my message would be crushing to her; it could only mean *cancer*. She'd already gone through a similar call many years before with my father. It was the phone call that changed all our lives.

Next I dialed my sister Holly, praying she'd be out, too. Once again God answered my prayer, reaching only Holly's answering machine, where I repeated the message. I couldn't bear to hear their immediate reaction. I wasn't strong enough yet.

My sister arrived home first and called me right away. She seemed to handle the bad news well and said she had already contacted her husband, who was out of town at an oncology conference, and he was taking the first flight back to Boston to get me an immediate appointment with the best breast cancer team in the city.

Amazingly, George had never had business in Boston before in all the years with his company, but that morning he had learned he was being sent there for the next two weeks, just where I needed to go for my second opinion. I contemplated how miraculous it was that George was being sent on this trip. But as usual, God was a step ahead of me all the way.

My mother's call came in next, and I almost hated to answer. I couldn't bear hearing the heartbreak in her voice, but after I said hello she spoke calmly. She was doing what I asked her to do, being positive and uplifting even in the face of this shocking news, Praise God. Still I knew in my heart she was devastated. I thought to myself, how powerful a mother's love! As we talked she reminded me how good God had always been to me, and how good He would continue to be in this latest affliction.

I asked her to call my sister Nancy, as I had to tell Joanna. I couldn't keep up this brave front much longer. She assured me she'd call everyone and prayers would be offered up everywhere.

George and I were drained from the devastating news, so we went to our bedroom to lie down. As I lay there in George's arms, our big dogs lovingly flanked our bed to provide their own source of protection.

Then I heard Joanna open the front door. I shuddered, wishing I didn't have to face this moment. It was her senior year in high school, and I wanted it to be memorable, but not like this. As she walked down the hall, I promised myself I'd be strong and minimize my diagnosis. I prayed for strength as her footsteps neared. She entered our room with a puzzled look as the dogs jumped up to greet her. George and I remained relaxed, welcoming her home as she sat at the foot of our bed. We asked how her day had gone, but she interjected, "Mom, did you get your results yet?"

"Yes, my results came in today."

She stared at me with concern. I continued softly, "Sweetie, the lab results revealed I have breast cancer. But don't worry. Uncle Robert will get me an appointment with the best breast cancer team in Boston next week. We'll leave on Monday for my second opinion."

I could see she was going with the flow. Since we were calm and accepting she did the same. I assured her I'd be just fine. We asked her not to tell her brothers should they call. In fact, they did call that evening, but I lied. I told them the results weren't back yet, and to drive safely on the trip home tomorrow.

Joanna and I did not feel up to attending the Valentines dinner, so I asked her to call her friend's mother to have her take over the leadership of it. Joanna would deliver the party favors and decorations to her friend's home close by. She left the house on her errand, and George and I felt she had taken the news quite well. Thankfully, I never saw sadness or worry in my daughter's eyes. She would do her utmost to never let me see it.

We learned years later that when Joanna arrived at her friend's house, she fell to the floor and sobbed uncontrollably, disclosing that her mother had breast cancer. Fortunately, her friend's mother was at home and comforted her by saying, "Joanna, your mother is so strong. If anyone can beat cancer, she can!" Perfect timing and perfect words that rang true to my daughter. She pulled herself together and returned home as if nothing had happened.

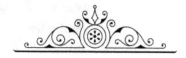

A Valentine's Day of Broken Hearts

Believers, look up—take courage.
The angels are nearer than you think.
Billy Graham

There are special days in life that stand out above the rest; Valentine's Day is one of those days for me. My grandfather loved Valentine's Day and taught us to love it, too, with his kind and generous spirit. How well I remember perching by the window at the foot of our staircase as my sisters and I waited for Gaga's car to turn down our street. In the kitchen our mother would be busy creating a warm and comforting meal and baking our favorite chocolate cake. Just when our wait seemed endless, his big shiny car made the turn, and we were jubilant to see what he had in store for us.

He always entered our house with his arms full, somehow making his way to the kitchen with three little girls wrapped around his legs. Then he stood before us, a hulk of a man in his business attire with his thick white hair and magnificent blue eyes that twinkled at our delight. He called our names to step forward and receive our special, individual gifts. Next came the Russell Stover chocolates, resplendent in their heart-shaped boxes and unforgettable to me to this day. Last but not least he swooped us up into his loving arms for a big bear hug and kiss, whispering in our ears how much he loved us.

In keeping with my grandfather's tradition, I wanted my children to have fond memories of Valentine's Day, too, so I made the day special for them, to include sweet stories of Gaga. Unfortunately, this Valentine's Day would be like no other we had experienced! Having to inform my sons of my diagnosis this weekend seemed like a cruel joke.

On Friday I left for work early, having barely slept a wink. Katy arrived shortly before me. By the looks of her puffy eyes, she had cried all night long, but ever efficient, she ensured that coffee and a muffin awaited me on my desk. We reviewed everything that needed to be done in the coming weeks when I would be absent, and she disclosed her concern for the company. I told her Ben had called, his voice clearly betraying his own concern. After assuring him I'd be fine, I urged him once again to speak to his uncle about assistance.

Later that day, after helping me to my car with the piles of paperwork I would complete over the weekend, Katy hugged me tight and warned that I shouldn't keep pushing myself in the midst of this frightening diagnosis. I told her that I needed to leave the office in good order, which would be one burden off me, giving me peace and allowing me to concentrate on myself. Even in the face of aggressive breast cancer I had to take care of the company we worked so hard to build. She understood.

As I walked into my house the phone rang. It was Ben, calling to say he'd been to see his uncle. My heart skipped a beat, and I held my breath as he gave me the news. After all these years of stress and strain, Ben had finally asked for the money!

I stood there dazed when he said, "You were right. I told him I needed to borrow some money and before I could go any further he got up from the table and wrote me a check."

"Did you explain everything to him?"

He replied, "I didn't have to. He was glad to help me."

I was incredulous. Apparently it took a cancer diagnosis for Ben to finally resolve the company's problem. I thought about how taxing these years had been on me. How many times I'd shown him, on paper, the promise of the future, and had told him the future couldn't arrive until we resolved the financial stranglehold that gripped us. Yet the resolution never came until all my health warnings took their toll, leaving me on a precipice.

I hung up from Ben and busied myself with prayers for our sons' safety in getting home and asking God for strength to tell them the troubling news. My older son, Merritt, was due home any minute. Blake would be along in another hour.

I was in the kitchen when Merritt arrived. Our big dogs greeted him first, with fiercely wagging tails. After working his way around them Merritt reached out for me and wrapped his arms around me. "Hey, Mama," he said, as he kissed me on the cheek. It seemed so good to hold my handsome, dependable son once again. How I wished I didn't have to tell him the bad news.

"Oh, Mom, did the surgeon's office finally call with your lab results?" My hand slid off his shoulder and down his arm. Taking his hand in mine, I took a deep breath and looked into his loving face.

"Yes, they called. Actually they called yesterday but I wanted to talk to you in person tonight."

"What's going on?" he questioned calmly.

I prayed for God's support. "It's breast cancer, son."

I watched for the emotional shock, but there was none. Merritt's face remained unchanged. I was thankful for his courage, needing him to react just as he did.

"Are they positive, Mom?"

"Yes, no question."

He quickly shifted gears, being the best cheerleader any team could ask for! "You'll be fine, Mom. You'll beat this thing." It was that simple. I watched him as words of encouragement spilled from his mouth, words I had spoken to him when life didn't go the way he hoped it would. He was good at it, convincing: a chip off the old block. I hugged him, assuring him God would take me through it as he'd taken me through everything else in my life.

Then I asked Merritt to make himself scarce when Blake arrived, wanting to break the news to him privately. He joined his Dad in the study, where I could overhear them talking about Marshall University football, a subject of endless fascination.

One more child to tell, I said to myself. But Blake, my other wonderful and handsome son, was also the most sensitive. Merritt and Joanna would hide their broken hearts, but Blake would wear his on his sleeve.

He walked in a short time later with his usual excitement about returning home. I hugged him warmly as the dogs wove around our legs. "Where is everyone?" he asked, as I pulled him into the kitchen. I could always count on Blake being hungry, and he sat down at the table as I pulled his favorite sandwich fixings out of the refrigerator. He updated me about school and friends, our conversation going back and forth, but just as I started to cut his sandwich in half, he suddenly asked if I had received the biopsy results. I put the knife down, took a deep breath, and turned to face him.

"Actually I spoke with the doctor yesterday, Blake. Unfortunately, the biopsy revealed I have breast cancer."

The shockwave came over him, like a boxer taking a blow to the head. I tried to be as casual as I could, explaining that I wanted him and Merritt to be home safely before I told them. His stricken look and the sadness in his eyes were almost too much to bear, yet I stayed the course, trying to make it easier for him. I placed the sandwich in front of him. He asked what the doctors told me about the diagnosis. I started telling him the details that I still didn't fully understand myself. Suddenly he shoved his plate out of the way and folded his arms on the table, put his head down and bawled. Through his tears he repeated over and over, "Mom, I can't lose you now, you're too important to me, I just can't lose you."

I wanted to cry, too, but I had to demonstrate that I would survive all that lay ahead of me. Sitting down beside him, I stroked the back of his head.

"Blake, you know Mama has a deep faith in God, He'll take me through this, you'll see, I'll be fine." I reminded him of all the stories I told him throughout his childhood, how God intervened in my life and healed me time after time. With my encouragement he slowly pulled himself together, wiping tears away with the back of his hand.

"So you're not worried, Mom?"

"No, I'm not. I'm going to put my hand in God's hand like I've always done, trusting Him all the way."

We chatted on as I urged him to finish his sandwich, making light of it all. I could see his gradual adjustment to this disconcerting revelation. Before long Blake's welcome home committee was at the front door, his old friends entering our house, excited to have him home for the weekend. They had no idea what had just transpired and coaxed Blake to go out with them. He looked at me quizzically, and with a wink and a smile I told him to run along and have fun with his buddies.

Moments later, after first saying hello to his dad, Blake and his friends were out the front door, laughing and calling each other names like old times. I shut the door and leaned against it with my eyes closed, thanking God for allowing my children to receive the dreadful news so well.

Saturday found us hanging out in the living room, making plans for Joanna to go to Marshall in the fall, putting on brave faces for each other. I had to get through this weekend and put my children's fears to rest. Somehow I put together a lovely meal for Valentine's Day, with heart shaped candy boxes, cards, and gifts laid atop the dining room table. But no one was in the mood for celebrating. We had always cherished sweet weekends with all of us together, but this was a weekend of broken hearts!

Sunday afternoon came too quickly, time for the boys to leave. They planned to follow each other back to school, each looking out for the other. I held them tight as we said our goodbyes, assuring them we'd get through this, reminding them to keep me in their constant prayers. I waved to them until their cars were out of sight. I hated to think of them driving over the icy roads ahead with this terrible news on their minds.

Back inside our house Joanna and I talked about the next two weeks of her being on her own while George and I were in Boston; her friends planned to take turns spending the night, and their parents would check on the girls from time to time.

I also had work to do for Ben that night before I left town. He called that evening to see how things were going, and I said I couldn't talk long as I was still hard at work making sure everything was in order for him and the company. He thanked me, saying I'd be in his thoughts and prayers.

As the hour neared midnight I finally accomplished what I had set out to do. These weeks of extra work were difficult considering the health issues that loomed over me, but now I was finished and it was liberating! Ben and the company would be safe. Even if I were away a month, he'd know what to do.

George and I headed to my office to drop off the work. He asked me to hurry, wanting us to get some sleep that night—our bags were packed and ready for Boston. He carried my paperwork as I unlocked the office door. We crossed the lobby to Ben's private office and placed my pile of devotion on his desk; instructions for keeping the business running smoothly topped my hard work. From my purse I pulled out a handwritten note, in which I told him not to worry about me. I reminded him of my faith and signed my name as I had so many times throughout the years, "Semper Fi, Cathy," invoking the Marine Corps spirit. Yes, 'Always Faithful' said it best.

George had gone back to the car to keep the motor running, as it was cold outside. I walked toward my office on the other side of the building, flipping on the light to my home away from home. My desk was covered with notes of support from our staff. Atop one of the notes was a small bottle with a note from our staff member Jean: "Some years ago I needed this water from Lourdes for something I was going through. Today I give it to you to use." I put her note along with the bottle into the zippered compartment of my purse; the note comforted me, and I was grateful for Jean's thoughtfulness.

I stood there looking around my decorated office, remembering the challenges I had to overcome to buy this building for Ben in the suburbs. I recalled our excitement, in the mid-1980s, on the day we moved in. I then ran my fingertips across the nameplate on my door as sadness consumed me, but I shook off my feelings and crossed the lobby to set the alarm. I only had a few minutes to vacate the property as I turned off the lights. The moon's glow filtered through the large windows of our office space as I walked to the exit door. I turned around, breathing it in one last time. It was a place I was truly proud of, having built it from mere dreams to a beautiful reality.

My heart was heavy as I exited the premises, but it was finally time to take care of me—something I hadn't done in a very long time!

Second Opinion

Quiet your mind, listen for the voice, do what feels right,
look for signs to direct you, and watch how
the coincidences and miracles start to happen.
Dr. Bernie Siegel

We made our way home in short order and climbed into bed. I was exhausted from the events of the past few days and quickly dozed off, but during the night a vivid dream began to play itself out.

I saw myself leaving the office again, heading toward my car, when suddenly I felt the overwhelming presence of others around me, and in a silent, surging motion, I was propelled toward a type of platform and a set of tracks. Around me were throngs of women. Some of them looked normal while others were baldheaded. They were somber and expressionless, but their eyes, like mine, telegraphed heavy burden. At this point I couldn't speak or react.

I heard the grating of steel on steel and saw a headlight hurtling toward me. With a screech a roofless carriage halted in front of me. A small door on its side opened automatically as a steamy mist arose from its underside. The first seat in the conveyance appeared to be a particular shade of blue: its color seemed familiar but I couldn't place it. Printed on the seat were three large letters in black, ABC, glistening in the moonlight, appearing wet. Reaching for anything that could make sense at this point, I thought these letters must be the name of the conveyance company.

I surged forward with the crowd and stumbled onto the floor of the front seat. I did not want to go on a ride and I protested loudly, "I need to go home." I stood up and regained my balance, but the small door to my side closed abruptly. With a forceful jerk I fell back onto the seat. I tried to move but found I was attached, as if glued, to the three large letters, ABC. I desperately tried to free myself, flailing in all directions, but no amount of effort broke me free. A force I had never felt before had me in its grip. With that the ride began and I became its prisoner.

I looked down in front of me and noticed the safety bar to my seat was gone! No bar, no seat belt, nothing to hold on to, and no way off!

The carriage quickly approached what looked like a tunnel with widely spaced walls and a far-reaching ceiling. The cavernous darkness terrified me. Only the tracks lay ahead of me now, echoing with steel on steel, but the carriage had slowed. I could see signs lit up ahead. Finally the message was distinguishable. I gasped in terror as I read aloud, "*THIS RIDE MAY BE HAZARDOUS TO YOUR HEALTH.*"

I glanced back to see if anyone else was on the ride, for surely this journey could not be meant for me alone. In the darkness I made out the silhouettes of many passengers, the women who had been on the platform and others. I couldn't see their faces, but their presence alone told me we were meant to be on this journey together.

The ride snaked its way slowly around a bend in the tunnel. Ahead I could now see many video billboards on either side of the tracks, looking like a continuous drive-in movie. One billboard introduced the story of a small child. I tried to quiet my mind and in doing so I recognized the little girl as myself! Shocked, my head swung from side to side as the video boards depicted each year of my life, taking me through chapter after chapter.

I desperately needed to get off this ride, but it continued to tug forward, heading deeper into the tunnel and picking up speed. The temperature dropped and I felt a chilling wind rush over my body, icy fingers of air raking across my face. The next billboard flashed: DANGER UP AHEAD. I saw scenes with doctors and equipment in them, people and places I didn't know, but I knew this was about my disease. I heard myself cry out in the tunnel, "Oh dear God, I had no idea this diagnosis was so frightening. How did it happen? Why has my body betrayed me? Please, dear God," I screamed, pulling my hands to my face, leaning forward, "I just want to get off this ride!"

In a sudden moment of clarity I realized I was no longer stuck to my seat. I tilted my body to one side, seeing the letters still there. I needed to remember them; tomorrow I would call the company, reporting the frightening ride I'd been forced to go on. But as I sat back down I felt something traveling through my being. It was ominous, journeying up through my insides, settling in my left breast. I felt sore and engorged.

I was also chilled to the bone from the speed we were traveling. Shifting in my seat again, I saw that the letters had now completely disappeared. And then the realization of what was happening hit me hard! "Oh my," I said aloud, "ABC—it means Aggressive Breast Cancer, and it has invaded my body with all its evil."

Fear gripped my being in a way I'd never experienced before. I couldn't get off the ride because it held me firmly in its grip, with no intent of letting me go. The carriage made a turn and we again plummeted down a long, steep hill. My heart was in my throat. If the ride hit a bump I would surely be thrown out onto the tracks. At the speed we were traveling I would surely die.

As the ride continued to rocket through the tunnel I had no choice but to try to calm my fears, no matter what the speed and the warning signs portended. I knew I needed to go to the place within me where God abides. He'd help me—He always had. "Concentrate," I said to myself. "Remember mother's words from childhood, "Go to God."

When the ride neared the bottom of the hill, by the grace of God I was still in my seat.

And then, another miracle, I thought I heard my husband's voice from somewhere behind me. George was shouting, "Honey, I'm here for you. We'll get through this together like we've gotten through everything else that's come our way. Sit tight and hold onto your faith, God will get us through." His voice filled the tunnel with conviction and determination.

I turned around fully then and saw my mother. She was trying to reach out to me but my carriage was too far from hers. I cried out pitifully, "Mama," just like I did as a child. She shook her head in disbelief. My eyes fixed on hers; I could see her fear and her pain. Her child was stricken with a dread disease, and she, too, would have to stay on the ride and see it through. The ride with its whiplash twists and turns, at speeds no ride dare travel at any amusement park. This ride had a mind and a power of its own.

My own children then raised their voices behind me, shouting energetically, encouraging me in the face of the chilling wind and their own fears. And they were soon joined, in what began as a cacophonous roar, but settled into a sustained and magnificent song of support for me, by the voices of my siblings, uncle, cousins, nieces, nephews, friends, neighbors—everyone whom I loved so dearly, here with me now, seeing me through this tunnel of darkness.

And then a feeling of desperation hit me as we passed another warning, this time the most ominous of all: "CONTINUE AT YOUR OWN RISK." What would happen to my family and friends on this ride? How good they were to come this far, but I couldn't let them die for me!

I knelt sideways on the floor of the carriage, looking under my seat, and found a lever with "Push to Release" printed on it. I had to free them, all of them, this very second. Using every bit of my strength I pushed the lever down and felt the rest of the train release and disengage itself, instantly losing momentum. My carriage broke free and sped on, careening under its own power. The light at the helm flickered wildly and then extinguished. I was now in utter darkness, but my loved ones were safe, and solace washed over me.

But the ride wasn't finished with me yet. The tracks became pitted and bumpy, the air was turbulent. The automated voice in the tunnel kept repeating, "Go back, go back. Dead man's curve up ahead." If only I could, I thought.

Common sense told me that my light carriage, at the speed it was traveling, would jump the tracks, and the ride would do what it had set out to do all along... kill me!

The tracks seemed high in the air now, and a hot, strong draft rose from a cavern below. One side of the carriage left the tracks as we continued round the curve sideways, throwing me against the opposite side of the seat. Shards of steel flew past me as the carriage began to shake itself apart. Sparks spewed out from the wheels, momentarily lighting the dark and infinite space. I peered down into the abyss, where I saw death calmly staring back at me, whispering my name, and coaxing me to give up.

At that moment I was given the grace to call out, "Dear Jesus, please give me your peace that surpasses all understanding. Help me know that you are with me, that I am not alone." I stayed in prayer, willing my mind to focus its entire strength on the glory of God. Just then the cold steel seat I was holding onto felt like fabric. The carriage bounced down hard several times, still shrieking, but then the change became unmistakable. Light filtered into the tunnel as my carriage journeyed upwards, and when I looked to my side, there was Jesus, and I found myself seated on His magnificent blue robe. All at once everything became crystal clear, and I knew without a doubt . . . He had been there with me all along.

The ride had been terrifying, but now I felt comforted in my dream state, wanting to remain there to hear what Jesus had to say. But at that exact moment, just before dawn, our alarm clock rang out intrusively, and we jumped out of bed and dressed quickly.

Before leaving I went to Joanna's bedroom to say goodbye. As she lay there sleeping, I kissed her softly on her cheek, whispering, "We're leaving, sweetie, have a good day at school and don't worry about me." She nodded with her eyes closed, as if to escape the reality of the moment. I turned to leave, stepping over the big dogs, who had moved into her room protectively.

As I reached the doorway Joanna spoke, her morning voice cracking. "I love you, Mom."

"I love you, too, baby girl."

As I looked back at my sleeping beauty, I whispered a prayer over her, believing God would see her through this difficult time. I could only imagine what was going through her mind. She'd just turned eighteen, and my diagnosis was forcing her to fast-forward into adulthood. We'd never gone away and left her alone in the house before, but in light of this crisis we had no choice. She'd be at college in six months anyway, and knowing she was a responsible child comforted me.

Later that morning we landed in Boston and headed to Holly's house in Concord. When we arrived, I could tell Holly was trying to keep her emotions in check, but she welcomed us warmly to her home. That evening after dinner, Robert discussed the appointments he was able to set up for the following day. I was grateful to have him as my brother-in-law.

Early the next morning George, Holly, and I went to meet with some of Boston's finest. My first appointment was with a leading oncologist at Beth Israel Hospital; he would head up my second opinion. I liked him immediately. He studied my sonogram, reviewing my doctors' reports. After he examined me, we all met with him in his office.

Holly took notes as the doctor told us about a specialized protocol at Lombardi Cancer Research Center at Georgetown University Hospital in Washington, D.C. He said that if the cancer hadn't spread I could go to Lombardi for what he called the cure, a course of treatment he outlined. He remarked that he had many patients with large localized breast cancers like mine who were still doing fine a decade after going through the treatment he discussed. He advised me that next week would be a week of testing.

Holly questioned, "So if the large mass hasn't spread, she has a chance?"

"Yes, that's right."

Holly continued, "Doctor, my sister wasn't supposed to see her gynecologist for another few months. What would have happened if she hadn't felt the change in her breast and simply waited?"

"We don't want to go down that road," he replied.

Just then I heard the words *Divine Intervention* emanate from my mouth, wondering where they came from. Immediately the doctor turned to me and said, "That's exactly right, hold on to those two words!" We shook his hand, thanking him for his time. He told me my next appointment was with the breast surgeon.

Later that afternoon Katy called with some business questions as well as to check up on me. She told me Ben wasn't working because he was having problems with his back; it looked like surgery was imminent. I thought how strange it was that the two of us had health issues at the same time! In all the years we'd worked together Ben never missed a day, so I decided to call him. When he answered, I could hear the pain in his voice as he asked how things were going.

I replied, "Sadly enough, the years of unrelenting stress have taken their toll on my health. Now that you finally have the money from your uncle, thankfully those burdens will be gone. Don't worry about anything, Ben, we'll get through this together."

In closing he whispered, "I love ya, Cath," which I repeated back to him. We were dear friends, going through the unexpected in life.

George had meetings the following day so my mother and Holly accompanied me to my appointment. Meeting the surgeon was an entirely new experience. After reviewing my x-rays, records, and lab tests, she proceeded to examine me, asking if I'd like to have my family present as she explained my findings.

I said I would, because by this time modesty was no longer an issue for me. My breasts were no longer for my husband to see or for the occasional time I wore a low-cut dress. Now they were mere specimens of science. The surgeon exposed my chest and invited my mother and sister in for a closer look, as she touched the area where the mass was hidden. She explained that it was large and deep in my breast tissue.

She then extended her index finger, gliding it over my left breast to the center of my chest, saying, "This is where her lungs are located. The proximity and size of the mass lead me to believe it may have already metastasized to her lungs." The upcoming tests would validate her conclusion, if this were so.

For some reason we weren't absorbing this new information. "What would that mean?" I asked, incredulous.

She continued, "If that's the case, I suggest you take a trip to a beautiful island somewhere."

Still bewildered, I asked exactly what she was talking about?

She replied, "For the limited time you would have left, you should go someplace nice and live out your days."

I got it! Of course I didn't believe her prediction, but I could see it unnerved my mother and sister. Somehow, every bit of bad or alarming news made me feel more and more like I was having an out of body experience; by God's grace I continued to stay calm.

Being back home in Massachusetts was something I always looked forward to. It meant time spent with family and enjoying great food from the sea. So no matter what was told to me, at the end of each day all I wanted was a big plate of fried clams! As my family looked ghostly white from all the frightening information, I could be found asking a nurse, a lab technician, or anyone at all, "What restaurant nearby makes the best fried clams?" My family wasn't hungry, but I was famished and looking forward to my plate of clams! To lighten the mood at dinner, I assured everyone that if any results came back bad (which I knew they wouldn't), I'd simply announce, "Time for fried clams!" It broke the tension and made everyone laugh, with me laughing the hardest.

However, a long weekend lay ahead of us with many unanswered questions. George finished up his work in Boston for the week, suggesting we head to my mother's on the South Shore for a change of scenery. Holly and Rob were looking for a summer home on Cape Cod and asked us to meet them at a beach community they were interested in. After a brief night's stay at my mom's, we headed for our rendezvous. Although we were happy to be there, the cold and blustery February weather hid the true beauty of old Cape Cod, with its summer months that I loved so dearly.

We drove through patches of snow and ice and met Holly and Rob in a town called Mashpee. They took the lead as we followed behind and turned into a community called New Seabury. George and I couldn't believe our eyes as we remembered taking Sunday drives in the late sixties to this unique area of California-style model homes. We had planned our life together, thinking we might settle in this new and different community one day. It had been our little secret, a location we'd almost forgotten about, and now here we were, standing in its midst under circumstances we never could have imagined.

Yet the day of house hunting turned out to be a great diversion and we loved the house they were thinking of buying.

On Sunday we were invited to Nancy's for dinner. It was good to see my niece and nephew again; their youth combined with their excitement at seeing us helped keep the day upbeat. After dinner Nancy's friend Cheryl came over, wanting to talk with me. We felt an instant connection. She took my hand and sat beside me on the sofa, revealing that years earlier she, too, had been diagnosed with breast cancer and wanted to support me during this unsettling time.

She went on to explain that she had a mastectomy and reconstruction years ago. She was whole again: my journey was just beginning. She asked if I wanted to see her reconstruction, and since I seemed to be headed in that direction myself, I said yes.

I knew she was sacrificing her modesty to put my mind at ease as we entered the powder room and closed the door. She unbuttoned her blouse to reveal her breast, which, surprisingly, looked completely normal. And in that intimate setting she quietly offered me words of wisdom that helped carry me through the adversity to come: "Cathy, you have a long road ahead, and I want to pass on to you the words that were given to me when my journey began." Then she simply said, "*Stay in the day.*"

A woman I'd never met before gave me an invaluable gift, four simple words to live by. Like so many busy people trying to manage a family, a business, and a schedule, I lived mostly in the future: next week, next month, next year. I seldom spent enough time in today. But with all that lay ahead of me in the months to come, trying to manage the future as I normally did would surely overwhelm me. I took her simple words to heart, now determined to stay in the day God gave me and not fret about tomorrow.

The next day Katy called, saying Ben's surgery went well. She was still upset, saying she couldn't work there without me, and then surprised me by saying she was applying for a new job. I begged her to reconsider but she was resolute. I sensed that she wasn't telling me the complete story, but we left it there for the time being.

Just before heading back to Boston on a chilly February night, we were in my mother's living room saying our goodbyes, when a frantic knock came at her door. When my mother opened it, there stood Nancy looking fearful as tears glistened in her eyes. I rushed to see if she was all right. She blurted out that Holly called her and conveyed that she had been running through her house in a hysterical state, crying, "Why Cathy, why her?" Luckily Rob was coming in from work and tried to reassure her.

Nancy continued, "Holly was inconsolable. She called to ask for everyone at my church to pray for you tonight during Bible study. I assured her I was going up to the altar to place you and your circumstance there." I thanked Nancy for her concern and prayers, saying I believed all would go well with the tests tomorrow, for my faith was strong. She stood there bundled in her winter coat, her brown eyes shining like glass as she fought back the tears. Then she stepped in closer and lowered her voice. Her lip quivered with emotion as she said, "*Cathy, you need to beg God for your life. Beg Him.*"

"But why would I beg Him? He has always been there for me."

In nearly a whisper she pleaded, "But this time your life is at stake. Tell Him you're young and you have children to raise, beg Him for more time here on this Earth." Her tone was desperate, and I assured her I'd think it over.

After Nancy left I looked to my Mother, who remained strong throughout everything. I sat down on the sofa between her and George as she patted my knee.

"The girls are frightened for you but your faith will see you through, just as it did when you suffered those horrific asthma attacks as a child. They were too young to remember all you went through and to see your great faith in God, but I witnessed it! Tonight as you go to Jesus, ask for His healing touch, knowing He'll heal you as He's done many times before."

She was unwavering, adding to my courage. George put his arm around me and said, "Honey, we're going to *stay in the day*, we'll get through this like we've gotten through all the obstacles in our lives."

We returned to Boston that night and George soon went to bed. I wasn't tired, so I decided to take my shower, saving time in the morning.

I took my purse into the bathroom with me and reached inside to find my comb, but my fingers felt something unfamiliar, a bulge in the side pocket. I opened the zippered area and pulled out a small bottle, realizing it was the bottle of water from Lourdes. I reread Jean's note as I set the bottle aside for the time being.

In the shower the warm water felt good as it caressed my body. As I soaped up, my hand glided over my left breast, which felt foreign to me now, seeming harder than it had been a week ago, harder and larger. I closed my eyes, turning my face up into the spray, trying to reach a different realm. Nancy's face came to mind, and I remembered her plea: "Just beg God, Cathy, please just beg Him!" Nancy had been in the medical field for many years. She still had many contacts at the local hospital, contacts she called close friends. Maybe one of them had told her just how dire my situation was?

I thought of what she had told us, imagining Holly running through her house, Rob finding her that way, trying to console her. I could see my mother at her front door as we left, assuring me I'd be fine, all the while her heart breaking. Then I thought about George lying asleep in the next room, exhausted from trying to run his business while simultaneously supporting his wife as she faced each new day of medical suspicions.

I thought of my recent phone conversations with my children as we drove to Boston. Joanna called, saying she was praying for me, and lots of other people were praying, too.

"You'll be fine, Mom, right?"

"Of course I will, sweetie."

Merritt and Blake called, assuring me they were praying constantly. Blake had said, "I'm so proud of you, Mom, proud of the way you've handled everything; you've been so strong and positive, I wanted you to know tonight how I feel." Hearing his words meant so much.

The water pulsated on me, relaxing my body as I went to prayer, talking to God like I would my dearest friend, someone to whom I could tell anything. Tonight I disclosed it all, recalling the terrible asthma attacks of my youth, lying there exhausted as I cried out for His help; He always came, healing me time and again.

Then I told God I wanted to see my children graduate from high school and college, see them marry and have children of their own one day. I wanted to grow old with my husband. I didn't want my mother or my children to suffer because of me. The more I implored God to heal me and sustain my life, the more emotional I became. Before long I was sobbing, pouring my heart out to my Heavenly Father and yes, pleading for His intercession.

Afterward, as I toweled myself dry, I picked up the bottle of water from Lourdes from where I had placed it on the counter. An image of the Virgin Mary was printed on the bottle, and although I'd never prayed to Mary before, I knew of her holiness, chosen among women to carry God's son on Earth. Over the years I had read articles about the healing waters of Lourdes; in fact, *The Song of Bernadette*, in which Mary appeared to Bernadette at Lourdes, was one of my favorite spiritual movies as a child. Coincidentally, Bernadette suffered from the same affliction I'd endured, asthma. Was this bottle of healing water predestined to come to me? The thought amazed me!

I opened the water as the room's humidity lay softly in the air, providing a heavenly ambience. I poured the water slowly into my cupped hand and massaged it into my entire body as I prayed, "Holy Mother of God, I ask that this healing water from Lourdes will heal me this night." The mist surrounded me as I continued to pour and rub the water all over my skin, knowing full well that tomorrow the CT scan would reveal all that was below its surface.

Hours later, as darkness still hovered over the city of Boston, our wake up call rang out, signaling the start of an intense day of testing. We arrived at Beth Israel Hospital where I was then taken to radiology. There, a technician injected dye into my arm to prepare for the CT scan. After I was positioned in the donut-shaped machine, the technician pointed out the small microphone near my mouth in case I needed her during the scan. The room was cold on purpose, and she placed a warm blanket over me just before leaving. I lay there on the table assessing my surroundings as a large black clock on the wall loudly ticked away the seconds. The CT machine began swirling at my feet with a loud droning noise. Looking up at the well-aged ceiling, I began to pray.

Once again I begged God for my tests to turn out right. I prayed that the large cancerous mass hadn't spread, and I asked for strength and peace. I was completely alone in the room, my very existence on the line, yet I feared no evil. And as I stared up in prayer, a miracle happened. Suddenly my inner thoughts and prayers ceased, and I knew unquestionably that I was in the presence of the Divine. He spoke my name and I listened as time and space stood still. A knowing poured over me, and in a flash of certainty I knew I would be fine. God continued His communication, "You will go on this journey, and at the journey's end you will write a book to give hope and inspiration to countless other women who will follow in your footsteps."

At the end of the brief encounter, I was abruptly thrust back into a noisy world, which seemed even louder after living in a Divine moment. I knew right then and there I was going to have a miracle! The peace of God flooded over me like the blanket that warmed my body. I lay there thanking Him for all He revealed.

The scan completed, a radiologist came out to speak with me. After introducing himself, he asked why a CT scan had been ordered. I summed up the events that brought me to Boston along with the surgeon's suspicions and asked him if he'd be kind enough to review my scans while I waited. He hesitated, explaining that a team of radiologists would scrutinize them later in the day. I told him I understood, but a preliminary look-see was of crucial importance to me. I implored him to take a look. He saw my beseeching eyes and said, "All right, but understand this is just preliminary."

He went to a hallway within my sight to view the images; my scans lit up on the light box. I watched as he studied each one in turn, whispering, "Dear Jesus, dear Jesus." Then he walked back toward me, as I held tight to God's promise.

He said, "Preliminarily speaking I only see a problem in your left breast. The mass is large, but it looks like it's just sitting there. Your bones look fine, too, but you'll still have to go for the bone scan to complete all your testing." I took his hand in mine and thanked him for his kindness, realizing it had been sent from God above.

I dressed and headed back to the waiting room, thanking God all the way, for His help and blessings. As I walked in, George saw me and came to his feet. I shared with him what God told me. Then I told him about the radiologist's preliminary findings. He hugged me tight and we were both thankful and relieved.

My next appointment was in nuclear medicine for the bone scan, where I was pleasantly surprised to find my family waiting for me in the reception area. I burst forth with my good news, although my mother wondered if my original diagnosis had been a mistake. I told her the radiologist said the mass was large but it hadn't spread, and more importantly God had spoken to me, letting me know I'd be fine. I also told everyone that one day I would write a book of hope and inspiration.

Not surprising to me, the bone scan I underwent that afternoon appeared to be clear, and I was told to expect a call from my lead doctor in the next few days, after all results had been fully analyzed. The call came on Thursday afternoon, when I was officially told the good news that the cancer had not spread. The doctor's voice was uplifted by my test results. In closing he said, "Now go to Georgetown for the cure."

He had offered me hope from the very beginning, and I would never forget his kindness and encouragement. As I would learn soon enough, however, not all doctors would offer me such hope! When I later spoke with the surgeon who had examined me, she seemed almost irritated by the oncologist's encouraging words, saying adamantly that no one can predict what my outcome would be. Yet every patient needs and deserves hope. Hope can turn a dismal diagnosis upside down.

Still craving fried clams, we went out for dinner to celebrate!

Later that evening, Katy called to check on my test results. I told her the good news as she praised God out loud. Finally, Katy could dry her tears, I thought. But life is never that simple. As she continued to cry she said it wasn't over my health at the moment, it was because Ben was letting me go! I sat down on the bed in my room. I was stunned, but thankfully, my mind was still in a higher place, focused on my many blessings. Whatever was going on back home, God had me on a new journey. He alone would see me safely through it all—that I knew for sure.

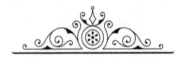

A Hard Lesson to Learn

For I know the plans I have for you, declares the Lord, plans to prosper
you and not to harm you, plans to give you hope and a future.
Jeremiah 29:11

We arrived home on Saturday afternoon and were excited to see our daughter and our big dogs again. Hugs and kisses went round our entryway. It felt good to be home after living out of a suitcase for two weeks, and we decided to stay in where it was warm, make a nice dinner, and enjoy being a family again. I told Joanna how proud I was of how she handled herself while we were away. The sweetness of her youth surrounded me as I said, "Sweet baby girl, God's giving us more time to make more beautiful memories."

But early on Sunday morning the big dogs sounded the alarm as a stranger approached our front door. Who would be here so early? George pulled on his pants and headed down the hall, trying his best to calm our fierce protectors as he opened the door.

"Is Cathy Davis at home?"

I sat up in bed and heard George say, "I didn't realize you delivered on Sundays."

"Yes, sir, we do."

George asked if he could sign, but the man insisted he needed my signature. I pulled on my robe, ran my fingers through my hair, and met George as he was coming to get me, saying it was FedEx.

He held the dogs as I signed for the envelope, thinking possibly it was from my doctors in Boston. But as I opened the outer wrapper another envelope was tucked inside, and I saw my name in Ben's handwriting, with "Personal" underlined. Inside was a formal letter from Ben, informing me I was no longer in his employ.

George asked me to read it aloud, so I did. In disbelief, I sat down on the chair in my hallway, reading the letter over and over to myself, unable to accept the fact that Ben sent this to me in the midst of my health crisis, or sent it to me at all for that matter.

After seeing the disappointment and shock on my face, George sat down beside me. He put his arm around me, pulled me close, and said, "For me this is an answer to a prayer." What was he talking about, I thought to myself?

But he continued, "I believe that everything happens for a reason, honey. Given your diagnosis, you will need all your strength to fight for your very life. But you are such a loyal person, I feared you would never be able to completely let your job go, which would put more stress on your ability to heal. But now with this termination letter, the decision has been made for you. Ben has set you free from your devotion to him and his company."

My husband knew me well; I would never have been able to let Ben down.

"But what about my salary?" I asked.

"It won't be easy without it, but we'll get through it somehow with God's help. Remember, we're going to *stay in the day!*"

Then George got up and took my hand and coaxed me back to bed to catch up on my sleep. But I couldn't stop looking at the opened letter on my nightstand, with Ben's cold signature, as tears streamed down my face, soaking my pillowcase.

Later in the day Katy called, wanting to get together, so we met at a nearby restaurant. It was so good to see her again, and she wanted to hear every detail of my spiritual encounter with God's communication.

I then handed her my termination letter. She shook her head regretfully. I told her I planned to call Ben in the morning to discuss what was going on. Suddenly, after the emotional roller coaster I'd been riding these past few weeks, topped off by a poorly timed termination letter, I broke down. Katy thought my tears were about my health issue, and she reached across for my hand, saying softly, "It's all going to work out, Cath, we'll stay in faith." But I shook my head no, trying to pull myself together. "I'm not crying about my health, Katy. I've come to realize that Ben and I will never be friends again."

First thing the next morning I called Ben, and he answered as if nothing had happened; he even sounded happy to hear from me.

I got down to business. "After all these years of being close friends, why in the world would you terminate me with all I've been going through? Can you imagine how difficult this diagnosis has been on me and my family?"

He answered straightforwardly, "I can only imagine the extent of treatment you have ahead of you, so I thought it best to let you go now."

I knew he was within his rights to let me go since Virginia is an "employment at will" state, and I knew full well that he would have sought counsel to substantiate his position before terminating me. He was also correct that I did have a lot ahead of me and he and his business needed to move on.

But I couldn't help feeling deeply saddened when I replied, "After all these years you let me go through a certified letter without any discussion about how we might get through this together?" I recapped all I'd done for him over the years, all the sacrifices I'd made. I reminded him where his company was when we first met. And now, because I had a health issue he was cutting his losses?

But I could tell his mind was made up. In a friendly tone he said, "It's all true, you helped me accomplish my dreams, and I'll always be grateful for all you did for me, but the time has come for us to go our separate ways regarding the company. Of course we'll still be good friends. You'll see, in a few months from now, once you're feeling better, we'll meet for lunch and we'll laugh about old times again."

I tried hard to keep my composure, but my voice cracked as I whispered, "Ben, you and I will never be friends again."

I thought about all the job offers I'd received during these stressful years, jobs in marketing, advertising, banking, and commercial real estate; the offers were flattering and lucrative but they meant leaving Ben in a terrible mess. My husband, children, and family urged me many times to get out from under the constant pressure I endured, but when I looked in my heart I knew I couldn't hurt Ben.

The disappointment I felt was smothering. Still he continued to talk in an upbeat fashion, but I was done listening. That's when I finally said, "Goodbye, Ben."

I knew in my heart it was a real goodbye, not just a farewell, but a severing of ties. Yes, Semper Fi had been my motto. Indeed, I was faithful to him and his company, even in the face of a life or death diagnosis. Unfortunately, in the midst of all I was going through, I realized how foolish I'd been to devote these years to Ben and his company, giving my all to something and someone who in the end could easily cast me aside. And the more I thought it over, I had to admit to myself—it was a hard lesson to learn!

However, like all things in life, everything does happen for a reason. We may not understand it at the time, but in time we will. I would come to realize that Ben played into God's master plan for my life. God had big plans for me, and without my knowing it then, I was headed in the direction of my Divine Destiny. And no man can keep you from that!

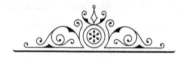

The Protocol

Life is 10 percent what happens to you
and 90 percent how you react to it.
Charles R. Swindoll

As we had discussed with my doctor in Boston, he recommended that I consider participating in a cancer research protocol if my test results were appropriate for it. A protocol would provide me with individualized attention, and the research based on my outcome would help other women in the future. The Lombardi Cancer Research Center of Georgetown University Hospital in Washington, D.C., forty-five minutes from my front door, had a protocol underway for aggressive stage III breast cancer. I realized Lombardi was the place God was sending me.

George and I arrived there on Monday morning, and we were ushered into a room where a doctor would examine me. Since Georgetown is a teaching hospital, the room was filled with students and other doctors. My breasts were once again put on display for the room of professionals to see as the doctor pointed out the tumor area and measured its size.

Afterwards George and I sat down as the doctor explained the Stage III Protocol, stating that the goal was to reduce the size of the tumor before surgery through three months of neoadjuvant chemotherapy. I nodded in agreement, having been told in Boston that if they operated before shrinking the tumor, a surgeon might have to go deep into my chest wall, making reconstructive surgery difficult at best.

The doctor continued, "Then you'll have surgery, which will most likely be a mastectomy, a follow-up chemotherapy, reconstructive surgery, and then possible stem cell transplant. When your immune system is stronger you'll finish up with radiation."

It would be a long haul, but I was certain they were going to learn much from this study, potentially changing the way women with aggressive stage III breast cancer were treated in the future, even saving lives. I was almost sold on signing up for the intensity of the protocol, which would require traveling to Lombardi for several biopsies each week and receiving a much stronger dose of chemotherapy to determine if higher doses could stop aggressive breast cancer cells in their tracks. Still, if it would help other women, it must be what I was predestined to do.

The doctor asked if I had any further questions. I thought for a moment and asked, "After completing all the treatments you've outlined, what will be my prognosis?" It was a question I hadn't asked anyone yet.

He answered by asking me a question: "Do you want to hear the truth about your prognosis?"

"Of course I want to hear the truth."

He said that in having stage III aggressive breast cancer, I had a high probability of it returning with a vengeance within two years.

I was blown away by this revelation. Part of me understood that this doctor was trying to be helpful by being upfront with me about the disease itself, giving me the odds I faced. But he didn't know me, nor how powerful my God was. Refusing to accept such discouragement, I jumped to my feet and shared with all the professionals in the room what God told me on the CT scan table at Beth Israel. That said, I then declared I was going to have a miracle, resolute in my faith.

Momentarily I thought about going back to Boston to be treated by my doctor there, someone who offered me great hope. George stood up and put his arm around me as he coaxed me back down in my seat. Then a small-framed, dark-haired young woman with brown eyes stepped forward, and she was introduced to me as the oncologist who formulated the stage III aggressive breast cancer protocol. She looked down at me, extending her hand, as I looked into her kind eyes, recognizing she was wise beyond her years. We formed an instant connection, and instinctively I knew I was in the right place, feeling it in my spirit. She would be my oncologist, and together we would change the face of stage III aggressive breast cancer treatment forever!

We moved to her office to talk, where she explained more details about the protocol—it would be aggressive, just like the cancer—and she handed me the paperwork to review. I signed it, trusting God it was mine to do. She then asked me to follow her to an area near her office where there was a phone on the wall. She called someone in another part of the hospital who monitored a control box containing cards with "Taxol" and "Adriamycin" (chemotherapy drugs) written on them. The protocol was a serious study, its rules followed precisely. To establish randomization, my doctor asked the monitor to select a card, and whichever name was drawn would be the drug I'd start with. The choice was witnessed and my name and protocol number recorded.

The doctor remained on the line, waiting for the drug's name. I prayed silently for them to pick the right one, the drug that would annihilate my mass yet be easier on me to start with. The randomization chose Taxol, which the doctor then described as being the more tolerable of the two (if that were possible). I was thankful for this so-called easier choice, at the same time reminding myself the ride would be rough regardless. This was still aggressive chemotherapy with aggressive side effects.

Every two weeks for the next six weeks I would receive Taxol, then Adriamycin for the same interval, followed by surgery in June. I was advised I'd lose my hair soon after the first infusion and gain between twenty to twenty-five pounds. I vainly thought, not me! I'm the woman who walks on the treadmill every morning and watches her waistline. I assured the doctor I'd keep my weight in check, but I was warned the chemo regimen included steroids, giving me little control.

The oncologist told me her hope was that the large mass in my breast would shrink by 50 percent, the protocol's overall objective and its criterion for success. She wanted to do a biopsy on me first to establish a baseline before any chemotherapy was administered. I agreed instantly, wanting to start as soon as possible to prevent the monster in my chest from growing any larger.

With the biopsy completed my first treatment was scheduled for Wednesday morning. George and I were up early to face the day, the day medical science would begin to kill the cancer inside my breast. I talked to God constantly, asking for His strength for all that lay ahead of me, knowing He was with me all the way.

After arriving at Georgetown Hospital, a nurse practitioner escorted me to a special floor where the protocol was being conducted. I was given a private room with bathroom, television, adjustable bed, and an easy chair for George to sit in. He had brought his laptop and cell phone with him so he could keep up with his work.

The floor nurse entered my room with an IV bag of Taxol, explaining that it comes from the bark of yew trees, and sixty pounds of bark were required to treat one patient. Imagine a treatment coming from tree bark!

This would be my introduction to the wonders of cancer research. The first treatment would be done intravenously, and then, to save wear and tear on my veins, I would have a port inserted in my chest for further treatments. The nurse told me the infusion would take several hours as she added some calming drugs to the mix.

The first few days after treatment were the worst, due in part to the higher than normal dose of chemotherapy the protocol called for. By the time I returned home I was feeling feverish and my bones ached. It seemed odd, feeling strange in my own body as weakness and chills came over me. Yet, it was definitely tolerable, as I trusted that the drug was destroying my tumor. Each night as I lay in bed after saying my prayers, I imagined the chemotherapy to be like little video-type piranhas eating away at my tumor. Visualization helped me gain a sense of control.

At my next biopsy, my doctor said I'd need a home nurse to take my blood several times a week; high-dose chemotherapy required my blood to be checked regularly for toxicity. My blood would then be taken to our local hospital and the results sent to Lombardi, the objective being to keep me away from the hospital during flu season. I remembered that the mother of one of Joanna's friends was a visiting nurse, and after a few phone calls to make the arrangements, she became my nurse, another angel on my path to healing.

My oncologist also advised me that I would lose my hair after starting chemotherapy, but for some reason the idea of losing my hair didn't bother me—after all, it would grow back. I was in God's perfect peace and that's where I planned to stay. The hair loss began on a sunny afternoon in late March. A cool breeze was blowing as George and I walked toward a store. I ran into an old acquaintance and George went on ahead while I visited for a moment. The woman had heard of my diagnosis, and I told her I was doing well and expected a full recovery. Just then the wind gusted and all the hair above my right ear became uprooted. The large clump floated in the air, right before our eyes. I touched the side of my head to confirm that my hair was gone! Recognizing what had just happened, the woman said goodbye, wishing me well.

I looked for George in the store while holding the right side of my head. When I found him, I walked up to him and pointed at my bald spot with a straight face. We both burst out laughing—that's all we could do! We quickly checked out and headed home. George placed a stool in front of the big mirror in my dressing area. He had already bought hair clippers to shave my head before my hair fell out on my pillow. I sat there as he gently shaved my head, coming face to face with my bald self. I have to admit, it wasn't too bad—I could handle it. The next day George took me to be fitted for a wig. *Stay in the day*, we said time and again.

No matter what happened, each day I awoke with gratitude, remembering to say "in all things be grateful." I thanked God daily for everything, especially His healing touch. Furthermore, I never allowed anything negative into my brain. I didn't look up information about cancer or mortality rates. In fact, I was given a leading book at the time about breast cancer, and after paging through some of the doom and gloom, I returned the book to the store. Instead, I read everything I could that was positive, spiritual, and uplifting, filling my mind with only healthy thoughts.

Truly Impressed

For assuredly, I say to you, whoever says to this mountain,
'Be removed and be cast into the sea,' and does not doubt
in his heart, but believes that those things he says will be
done, he will have whatever he says.
Mark 11:23

My next appointment was at Georgetown University Hospital, where I would have a port inserted in my chest, which would make infusions much easier on me in the future. I was to have a biopsy the following day. The night before my biopsy, as I lay in bed in deep prayer, my hand passed over my left breast. It no longer felt hard and taut; in fact, it almost felt normal. Continuing my talk with God, my fingers pushed deep into the area where the tumor was located. I had received only one round of chemotherapy, but incredibly as I probed, my tumor seemed smaller.

I wondered if this could just be wishful thinking, yet I knew what I was feeling: the tumor was now half its original size. Such a reduction was the protocol's overall objective—but not after just one treatment! Yet I knew the mass was disappearing. I lay there in the darkness with George beside me in deep slumber as tears of gratitude filled my eyes. God and I were one. He was at work in my body, healing me once again.

As my prayer continued, I shared I had an appointment in the morning with my doctor, praying, "Dear Heavenly Father, I ask that tomorrow when my doctor examines me, she, too, will feel the difference and will speak the words 'truly impressed' to describe the miraculous change." I don't know why those precise words came to my mind, but they did. My doctor's confirmation would prove that my healing was taking place, as I witnessed the miracle unfolding in my life.

The next day as my doctor came through the door she greeted me warmly, asking how I was tolerating the high dose chemotherapy. I told her I was doing well, without mentioning the side effects, and she smiled as if to say, "I admire your attitude." I didn't tell her about my discovery. I was excited to hear what she would say, but I wanted her to do her own examination first.

She stood to the left of me and examined the normal tissue of my right breast. Then her trained fingertips went to my left breast. I watched her face above me as she looked through her glasses, concentrating as her fingertips probed the tumor site. I could see the astonishment in her eyes, yet I said nothing as she turned to refer to my chart. After her review she reached for the measuring gage: the true test of size and change. Her enthusiasm was evident, saying, "Cathy, your mass last week measured eight-and-a-half to nine centimeters, and today it measures four-an-a-half to five centimeters." She was elated; after all, I was in her study. She then leaned over me, closing my gown, and said,

"Cathy, I'm truly impressed by this change, after only one treatment of Taxol!"

I gasped, and grabbing her forearm, I said, "Doctor, while in prayer last night, I felt the tumor area and realized it was half its original size. I asked God for you to say precisely the words you said, confirming He's at work in my body."

She maintained eye contact with me and, after pausing for a moment, said, "Those were the only words that came to my mind." She then asked if she could invite the other doctors from the protocol to witness this amazing change; I agreed as she went to collect them. I lay there thanking God for my healing; the doctor had spoken but God gave her the words, the same words He'd given me! The beauty of the moment was so spiritual that it took me to higher ground.

The other doctors examined me also, and they, too, were "truly impressed," as my chief doctor stood there beaming. Once everyone left the examination room she performed another biopsy. Afterwards I reminded her of our first meeting when I told all the doctors in the room that I was going to have a miracle! She smiled at me as I placed my hand on her shoulder.

Looking her in the eye, I asked, "In medical terms, what would a miracle be called?"

"A CCR, Complete Clinical Recovery," I heard her say.

"Has it happened yet in your research?"

"No, it hasn't."

"Then I will be the first," I said with confidence.

When I returned home that day, I called or sent e-mails to everyone I knew, giving them the exact medical terminology for their daily prayers concerning my healing. Family asked friends and neighbors to pray; in turn, friends asked their friends and families to pray. Our military friends all over the country were praying. I was placed on the prayer list of many churches. Who knows, you may have prayed for me, too?

Shortly after my next chemotherapy, the mass just seemed to disappear. My doctor was unable to perform any further biopsies, and at my next doctor's appointment, no one could feel my tumor any longer. I was now advised to consider a lumpectomy after finishing the chemotherapy portion of the protocol, and if the pathology showed more cancer and lymph node involvement, a mastectomy would be scheduled for the following week. I agreed with the plan. Only months earlier I had been advised to have an immediate mastectomy, and now the large tumor was no longer palpable!

Time raced by, and I finished the three rounds of Taxol. I moved on to Adriamycin, a chemotherapy drug made from a bacterium that produces a red pigment. I'd seen the bright red bags in other rooms on the protocol floor. Since the bags looked like bags of blood, I decided not to think of them as toxic. Instead, I looked on them as the blood of Jesus, washing away my cancer cells.

I did have a harder time with the side effects of this drug, however. Adriamycin created uncomfortable sores in my throat, and I lost interest in all food except steak, mashed potatoes, La Croix Sparkling Water, and smoothies. God bless Joanna. Each day she brought me a Pina Colada smoothie to soothe and refresh me—it was my remedy, along with my pillow-top mattress! Once home after treatment, I always headed for my bedroom haven, where I indulged my fondness for Oprah Winfrey, flanked by my two big dogs, my faithful sentries.

At one of my remaining infusions, Jenny, the research nurse of the protocol, walked me from the Lombardi Center to my hospital room at

Georgetown, where she sat down beside me on my bed. Jenny was truly one amazing woman and revered by all. She made going through cancer as easy as it could possibly be in so many ways for all of us. As we sat there chatting while waiting for my treatment, I reminded Jenny with great conviction that I was going to have a miracle! She looked at me and said softly, "I believe you."

I realized at that moment that I knew nothing about her, except that she was always there for me. I then asked her if she was married and if she had children. She disclosed that she had been married for many years and they had tried everything to have a baby, but all efforts had failed. Instinctively, I reached over and laid my hand on her leg. I told her to ask everyone she knew to pray she would get pregnant. I said that I would start praying immediately.

But more importantly, she needed to believe she would have a miracle, even though she was almost forty years old! I could see the sadness in her eyes, and I knew that not being able to have children was an emotion-filled topic for her. As she left my room I called out, reminding her to simply believe!

Sometime not long afterwards, Jenny learned that she was expecting. Ultimately, she had two boys, proving once again that miraculous events happen every day, if only we believe!

The Presence of Angels

It's not whether you get knocked down; it's whether you get up.
Vince Lombardi

igns of spring were in the air; new life was all around me as I sat on my deck thanking God for it all. I kept my mind busy, planning Joanna's June graduation. I had paid for a party site back in January before my diagnosis. Given my health issues it wouldn't be the grand party I imagined, with a caterer and all the trimmings, but it would still be memorable. My family would help plan the menu and prepare the details.

During this time I had also had a short but fun experience participating in a Nightline story. The Lombardi Center had been asked if a patient could be filmed in the background receiving chemotherapy while the narrator described a new drug called Herceptin, which the FDA had recently approved to fight stage IV breast cancer. When asked if I could be filmed, I happily assented, knowing that any awareness I could bring to breast cancer treatment was part of God's plan. Unknown to me at the time, my brief connection with the Herceptin story would link me with another breast cancer patient in the future, a woman who would become one of my dearest friends.

In the meantime I had another appointment at the hospital, but on the appointed day I awoke with excruciating pain in my neck and jaw. The pain was so bad I could barely stand up, so George dressed me, put my wig on my head, and gingerly helped me to the car. I kept my hands pressed against my neck and jaw, trying to eliminate any jostling. The ride to Georgetown was grueling, the slightest flaw in the road making me wince. By the time we arrived, I was in pure agony.

At the front desk, we asked the receptionist to call my oncologist immediately. I was taken directly to her, and after she examined the area, she promptly called radiology. I was whisked away for ultrasound. When I returned to the clinic, the doctor saw me right away. She took a deep breath and explained I had three large blood clots lodged in my jugular vein; they were being thrown off by the port, and their size and location were quite dangerous. If the clots dislodged before they could be treated, they would likely cause a stroke and could kill me. She was admitting me to the hospital for an indeterminate time.

The port needed to be removed as soon as possible, but the problem was how best to do this, given the serious condition I was in. A nurse moved the wheelchair I sat in to the hallway while I waited for a hospital room. Thinking about a hospital stay weighed heavily on my mind, knowing that Joanna's party was coming up fast and nothing had been prepared yet. In my weakened state, I began to cry. The nurses knelt round my chair trying to comfort me, but I was inconsolable, sobbing even harder. The doctor was told of my crying and she left her office to soothe me, saying she had never heard me cry before. Kneeling down in front of me, she looked up into my face and assured me everything possible would be done to resolve this latest health crisis.

I took a deep breath and said, "Doctor, my daughter graduates in a few weeks. I have so much to attend to for the celebration, I don't have time to be in the hospital." The doctor stood up, patted my shoulder, and said, "I should have known she wasn't crying for herself. She's worried about her daughter's graduation party." Hearing her say it aloud made me see how silly I sounded in the midst of this extremely serious problem. I couldn't help but smile, making me laugh, along with everyone else. The mood lifted and my room was ready. I found myself lying in a hospital bed with three blood clots lodged in my jugular vein.

Later that day, the surgeon whom I had met earlier to discuss the surgical portion of the protocol came to visit me. He had heard about the clots and wanted to discuss the way forward. He and I had formed an instant rapport when we first met, so I already knew I could trust whatever he was going to advise. Greeting me warmly, he sat on the edge of my bed, saying he had just finished his last surgery of the day. He reviewed my chart along with the radiologist's report.

He said we definitely needed to take out the port, and I told him I wasn't afraid, but I had to be awake during the procedure. I did not want anesthesia, given the severe nausea it always caused me. He agreed conditionally, stating his own terms: I'd have an IV inserted, and if I felt any pain after my chest was numbed, I'd be given anesthesia to put me out. I agreed.

Later on my oncologist came to see me, telling me she was glad I was having the surgery in the morning. By this time, we were good friends. I was a guinea pig in her protocol, a case she was studying. She was the mind and hands of God to me. After all, God sent me to her: the creator of the universe preordained our relationship. I knew this doctor respected my unwavering faith. I admired her intellect combined with her kind and understanding demeanor, feeling blessed to be a part of her study.

The next morning I went to surgery, and the operation was a success without anesthesia. I was then put on blood thinners to shrink the clots and would need to give myself shots when I returned home. In the meantime I would stay in the hospital until the doctors felt the clots had shrunk enough for me to be out of imminent danger. The doctor assigned to my floor told me as long as I was in the hospital my insurance would cover the cost of the blood thinner, but once I was an outpatient he was skeptical the drug would be covered, adding it was quite expensive. He reminded me how serious my situation was, how close the clots were to my brain. If my insurance didn't cover the drugs, he couldn't release me before I was due to have breast surgery, the next step in the protocol.

Just to think I might have to stay in the hospital and miss my daughter's graduation was inconceivable. I asked the doctor if I could call my pharmacist while he was present to clarify the issue right away, and he agreed to wait. By now I knew the pharmacy number by heart. I prayed silently for my release as I dialed and asked to speak to the pharmacist. I told her of my situation, asking if she could look up my coverage for the expensive drug. I heard her typing on her computer, and then she said happily, "Yes, the drug is covered under your plan." I was elated and asked her to hold momentarily as I relayed this to the doctor. He looked surprised and asked to speak with the pharmacist himself for confirmation. Afterwards, he reluctantly decided to discharge me.

George happily came to get me, driving straight to the pharmacy to pick up my prescription. When we arrived, the pharmacist came to the window and apologized profusely, saying she'd somehow made a mistake. The drug wasn't completely covered (as the doctor had feared), leaving a large amount for us to pay. Yet, I couldn't be upset, as her error allowed me to go home, my prayers answered. The blood thinner continued to shrink the clots as the days at home went by.

At the beginning of June, Joanna's graduation party came off without a hitch. It was a family effort, with everyone pitching in to help with shopping, cooking, and preparations. I knew my limits at this point and was grateful for the help. In addition to our local guests, many old and dear friends arrived from around the country, to include Joanna's best friend, Carolyn, who had moved with her family to California years earlier. Mina even came in from Canada; after all, Joanna was her baby, too! The disc jockey kept everyone dancing all night long, and it was a wonderful celebration.

My former employee Jean arrived late, holding a plain rectangular box in one hand and a card for Joanna in the other. This was the woman who had given me the water from Lourdes. She had just returned from the annual retreat she attended in southern Virginia, where participants take a vow of silence for three days to commune solely with God. Year after year, Jean, who is a small-framed, soft-spoken woman, looked forward to the spiritual experience. She whispered in my ear that the box was for me, saying with a sweet smile on her face, "God spoke to me during the retreat. I finally heard His voice." I looked at her in amazement, thinking how angelic she appeared.

I could see she was moved by her experience as she continued, "The last day of the retreat, as I walked from my dormitory to the church in prayer, a picture of an angel captured my attention and I stopped to admire it. Just then the silence around me was broken. God spoke my name and said, 'Jean, before you leave today you must obtain this picture for Cathy Davis and give it to her just before her surgery.' I've waited all my life to hear God's voice, and when He spoke His message was for you."

The celebration and noise continued all around us but I was captivated, listening only to Jean. She continued, "When the retreat ended I went back to the hallway and took the picture off the wall. I took it to a priest there, telling him what you were going through and that God had spoken to me."

I stopped Jean, asking if she had been thinking of me or praying for me as she walked the long corridor to the church, but she shook her head no. She said the priest was moved by her story and he told her to do what God directed. The priest then insisted on blessing the picture at the altar. Jean continued to whisper in my ear, "So Cathy, God wanted me to give this gift to you; I simply followed what He told me to do."

Mesmerized by her words, I slowly removed the cover from the box. Inside I saw a beautiful angel gazing at a white dove as it landed in her hand with outstretched wings. A verse at the bottom of the picture said

Presence of Angels
The very presence of an angel is a communication.
Even when an angel crosses our path in silence,
God has said to us, "I am here. I am present in your life."

Emotion engulfed me as I stood in awe of God's communication. I had held tight to God's promise, contrary to many expert predictions. But even today, two days before my surgery, God found a way to speak to me. He had chosen Jean, a spiritual vessel, to deliver another message of hope. Praise Be to God!

After many of our guests had left for the evening, our family began to sing. The highlight was my sweet Uncle Donnie, coached by Joanna, singing "What a Wonderful World." I hadn't shared with them yet what transpired between Jean and me. I just stood there holding my new picture with God's message, as my heart, mind, and spirit filled with thanksgiving for this most special evening.

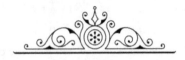

God's Promise Revealed

What you receive is directly connected to what you believe.
Joel Osteen

arly Sunday morning the girls left for beach week. Waving goodbye, I was glad Joanna was getting a break from cancer! My lumpectomy was scheduled for 8:00 a.m. Monday morning. Our guests were leaving, but my mother and Holly stayed on to accompany us. George decided the four of us should spend the night at a hotel near the hospital and have dinner at the restaurant overlooking Washington where we had celebrated many an anniversary. My last chemotherapy had been a few weeks earlier, and food was starting to taste good again. As we arrived for dinner we tried hard to keep the conversation light, discussing the recent party.

We enjoyed the meal and the city lights twinkling in the distance. When it was time to say goodnight I hugged and kissed my mother and sister, and they assured me I'd remain in their constant prayers. I felt good knowing they were doing so well, but years later Holly would reveal that when they closed the door to their adjoining room, they went to their beds, crying their hearts out into their pillows, fearing I'd hear them. They were saddened by what I had gone through, and desperately wanted my surgical results to confirm a CCR.

The new surgical plan called for making an incision at the original site of my tumor above my nipple. Whatever remained of the tumor and tumor bed would be removed, along with my sentinel lymph node and ten random nodes under my left arm: this would be an aggressive approach, providing pathology with a good amount of tissue sample to check for further cancer.

Morning came too soon and before I knew it I was signing in at the hospital. George hugged and kissed me goodbye, saying he was going to pick up my family. An orderly appeared with a gurney, taking me to the surgical ward. Just before the anesthesiologist administered my cocktail, I spoke to God, telling Him I believed in the miracle He'd given me, surrendering myself to His loving care.

The next thing I knew, a nurse was calling my name as I awoke to severe nausea and vomiting. The rest of the day found me sitting very still, trying not to move in hopes of preventing the room from spinning out of control. George sat there with me hour after hour, his presence comforting me. My mother kept checking on me, but Holly, who shares the same sensitivity to anesthesia, couldn't bear seeing me that way.

By early evening the anesthesia finally wore off, allowing me to be released. Drainage tubes had been inserted in the incision under my arm, running down my side and into a sealed plastic catchall attached to a belt at my waist. George was given instructions for how to care for me. Yippee, surgery was now behind me! When we arrived home the dogs ran to greet us, as always. Home never looked so good, my king-size bed beckoning to me. My family stayed until Thursday morning, the day of my check-up with the surgeon.

The doctor removed the surgical bandages carefully, replacing them with sterile ones. By the way he was talking I knew he was pleased with my progress. I had asked him before the surgery if I could accompany George on a business trip to Arizona slated for the end of this week. He said if I was feeling well and my incision looked good, he'd allow me to go. However, if pathology revealed more cancer, I'd need an immediate mastectomy the following week. I had agreed to his terms.

Now I asked, "So do I get to go on the trip?"

He gave me a thumbs-up, but also reminded me that pathology was still working on my tissue sample. I smiled and said, "Doctor, remember, I'm not going to need a mastectomy, I'm going to be the first CCR in the protocol." Everyone I knew was aware that pathology had my tissue sample; friends and family all over the country were saying prayers. He patted my arm and broke out in a big smile, saying, "Get out of here and enjoy your trip. Either way I'll see you next week."

George and I were thrilled with the green light, allowing us to go away. We headed home to pack, as we were leaving in the morning. I called my loved ones, telling them the good news, and closing each conversation with, "Keep praying for a CCR."

The next morning we hurried to catch our plane to Arizona. I was happy to be finished with aggressive chemotherapy, happy to once again be going on a trip with my husband, but more important, I was simply happy to be alive! To see us we looked like any other couple going on a trip, even though a wig adorned my bald head and my shirt hid the drainage tubes taped to my body. No one could guess all I'd endured during these past months.

We boarded the plane and found our seats. When we sat down we just looked at each other, knowing without a word spoken we'd made it through it all… together! Then George took my hand and squeezed it three times. As the plane climbed high into the sky, I returned our hand signal: the three squeezes meant "I love you." It had been our unspoken communication since we were young teenagers, riding the bus to school.

I lay my head back and closed my eyes, recalling another airport, years earlier when we were newly married. George was in the Marine Corps, leaving for Viet Nam. When the airline announced final boarding, we had said our long goodbye; there were no words left to say. We just stood there holding hands, not knowing if we'd ever see each other again. I squeezed George's hand three times, in return he squeezed mine, and then he turned to board his plane, headed for war.

Other memories came flooding back. Lying on a delivery table, trying desperately to birth our child, my body wracked with pain, clutching George's hand as the baby's head crowned, our world turning from peril to pure joy, George squeezing my hand three times. And so it was… whenever words would not suffice, our hand signal revealed the feelings in our hearts.

Now we were on a plane to some time alone. We could go out to dinner again and simply be normal for a little while. I could sit by the pool in the warm sunshine of Scottsdale, surrounded by God's majesty in every direction. I looked over at George and smiled excitedly. I felt like a bride on her honeymoon. I felt free for the first time in many months. Free to be me, not a patient, free to be a couple again.

We stayed at the Saddleback Mountain View Resort, near George's business meetings. Our suite was lovely, with large windows and all the comforts of home. Each new day in Arizona was spectacular. I sat near the pool in the shade, watching families at play, carefree vacations that in the past I'd taken for granted. I appreciated life as I sat there, surrounded by the beauty that God provided, thanking Him as birds flew overhead and the gentle breeze kissed my cheeks, all the while holding on to God's promise. There would be no mastectomy for me, I told myself; only good news awaited my return. I believed it with all my being, holding tight to God's mighty hand.

When George finished work for the day we went sightseeing, took walks, and had coffee at nearby cafés—even coffee tasted good to me again. The days flew by and on our last night we decided to have dinner at the resort's lovely outdoor dining area. George looked handsome in his new Ralph Lauren shirt as hand in hand we walked to the restaurant, sitting on the patio where we could view the grounds and the pool. Candles and torches surrounded us as stars twinkled above, while the moonlight added its own ambiance to the night.

George asked when my results would be in, and I said I really didn't know, but my oncologist had the number at the resort in case she needed to speak to me. He smiled, winking at me from across the table. We never spoke of anything negative. We focused on the night and our life together, enjoying our romantic evening as we stayed in the day, believing in God's message. After a sumptuous dinner we walked back to our suite. The moon was so bright we decided to sleep with the heavy drapes open. Only the sheers were closed, allowing the moon's illumination into our room. George kissed me sweetly as I turned and curled into him. He pulled me close and placed his arm around my waist, his fingers resting on my forearm. The moonbeams reminded me of my childhood, the nights when the asthma attacks were so severe and no air would come— the nights I called out to Jesus in desperation, and He answered the prayers of that little girl.

I closed my eyes, lost in those memories, as I prayed, "Dear Heavenly Father, I know you have been with me throughout this ordeal. I pray that the pathologist's report will come back soon and that the letters CCR will be told to me. I thank you for my healing and the miracle you've given me, in Jesus' precious name I pray, Amen."

It was late by the time I finished my prayers. I opened my eyes to the ambient light that seemed to embrace us as we lay there together,

George's rhythmic breathing comforting me, making me sleepy, too. Just as I started to doze off, his fingertips softly tapped my forearm three times. A feeling of love and contentment flooded over me as I drifted off to a deep slumber.

In the morning George left early for a final meeting without a sound. I awoke to the phone ringing noisily on the nightstand; startled, I opened my eyes to a sun-filled room. It was just before 9:00 a.m. I answered, still half asleep, my voice cracking from being unused. Someone on the other end called out my name, "Cathy? Hello, is this Cathy Davis?" It was my oncologist, and her voice was elated. She continued with great joy in her voice, "Cathy, you did it! You had the first CCR!"

I asked her to repeat what she had just said. Exuberantly she reiterated, "Cathy, you had a CCR!" Then she added, "There'll be no mastectomy for you. Enjoy the rest of your vacation, we'll see you when you return."

I was spiritually overcome and sat up in my bed, trying to digest the news. Rays of sunshine poured in and emotion overwhelmed me. Looking up I cried out to Jesus, my voice cracking as I humbly thanked Him and my Heavenly Father for the healing I'd been given. Rocking back and forth, I cried aloud words of praise: "My cup runneth over."

My heartfelt emotion turned to excitement, as I wanted to tell everyone about my miraculous outcome. The message God had communicated months earlier had now been validated by science!

Praise God from whom all blessings flow!

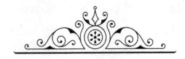

The Gift of the Word of Knowledge

Fear not, for I am with you; be not dismayed for I am your God.
I will strengthen you. Yes, I will help you. I will uphold you
with my righteous Right Hand.
Isaiah 41:10 (ESV)

*O*ur idyllic vacation came to an end, and we headed home. Peering out the jet's window into the infinite blue abyss, I thanked God for my healing. I was whole again. Once home I promptly called the Lombardi Center to make my follow-up appointments. A woman answered, asking for my name, and as we chatted, still on a high, I couldn't help but share my incredible results.

Excitedly she replied, "Oh my goodness, you're the woman who had the CCR?" I asked how she had heard about me and she explained that she didn't know my name, but the hospital was abuzz about a woman's remarkable response in the protocol. I said the medical community calls it a CCR, but I call it a miracle! She said she was inspired, hoping to meet me in person one day, making me realize that everyone thirsts for good news, especially in the cancer center of a hospital. As she made my appointments I smiled, thinking how my outcome would affect others, knowing the hope they, too, would receive.

I looked forward to seeing my doctors; I knew they'd be excited to see me, too. My success was their success as well. My first appointment that week was with my surgeon. He walked in to the examining room, grinning from ear to ear; I was grinning, too. He gave me a big hug, then he stepped back again and looked me in the eye, saying, "Well, you and the Big Guy did it!" In celebration, we burst into joyous laughter.

He examined the surgical site and said the area had healed nicely; a small incision scar would be all that remained. Finishing up, he said with a smile, "Cathy, your incision looks great! You said from the beginning, you wouldn't need a mastectomy, and it turns out you were right!"

My next appointment was with my oncologist. As I gave my name at the receptionist's desk, a staff member came forward smiling, introducing herself as the person I spoke with earlier to make my appointments. After hearing my miraculous story she wanted to meet me in person. I again thought about how much the human spirit yearns for good news.

As I walked the hall to the doctor's office, nurses came out to congratulate me as if I'd achieved celebrity status. When the doctor arrived, our excitement bubbled over as we embraced happily.

I had told her at our first meeting that God already knew my result. She had admired my faith, but she lived by scientific evidence: evidence that was now recorded in my chart. Our joy filled the room as she examined me.

After our short celebration, she then reminded me I would still need a follow-up cycle of chemotherapy in late July as part of the protocol. As we said our goodbyes I realized I wouldn't see her for well over a month, seeming odd to me since I'd seen her every week since the beginning of March. As I walked out the Lombardi Center's front doors, I was grateful for my life and the many blessings I was given.

George and I headed back home, our sunroof open as we rode along. The sun's rays embraced me as I stared out my window, realizing a summer of healing lay in front of me. My time was my own again.

The next morning I was outside on my upper deck, enjoying time off from the rigid hospital schedule, basking in the warmth of a summer's day. Lushly blooming flowers filled the planters that rested on the deck's railing, and I watched as beautiful butterflies landed amongst them. George had hung bird feeders in the branches surrounding the deck so I could enjoy nature up close, and birds of every description swooped in for their share of the goods.

While taking in all of God's handiwork, I realized that I'd never sat out on our deck for any length of time, due to the years of my demanding job. We had the deck specially designed and built years earlier, and although it was lovely, I was always too busy to enjoy it, until now! Shaking my head in regret, I realized all I'd missed. I was thankful for the new day and the new life God had given me.

Weeks earlier I had been warned by survivors as well as medical professionals about a down time after surgery, a time when a survivor isn't followed as closely as before. I was told it might feel like a safety net was pulled out from under me, no longer being protected by my doctor's watchful eyes. I thanked them for their warning, but I was confident this wouldn't happen to me, and I knew that to be true this very morning.

However, in early July when Holly called for our usual morning chat to ask how I was doing, her voice cracked as she said, "Cath, you were really lucky, you know. I've talked to people about your stage of breast cancer and they can't believe your results. We even know doctors who think your outcome was nothing less than remarkable!"

I replied, "But you always knew I'd be fine, right?"

"The truth is, you were so sure of your healing, you made us all believers." Surprised, I realized my family didn't believe I'd be fine; instead, I had convinced them through my faith.

Later that morning I had another call, this time from an old friend from our Marine Corps days. She checked on me regularly, reporting my progress to the people at her large church, where I remained on the prayer list. This friend is full of life—the mere sound of her voice can brighten any day. I asked her to thank the good people of her church for keeping me in their prayers.

Then she said, "Cathy, you don't sound like your cheery self, is everything okay?"

I shared with her my sister's words. She responded, "I can relate, as many times when I've explained your diagnosis, people were deeply concerned for you. I could tell they felt a miracle was the only thing that could save you."

"But you knew I'd be fine, right?"

She answered, "I prayed for you constantly, as well as everyone I knew, placing you in God's loving care. I knew He'd take care of you, but truthfully, it was your faith and attitude that convinced us you'd have a miracle."

Checking my watch, I thanked her for her faithfulness, saying I had to run as I was meeting George for lunch. I quickly pulled on my favorite wig, applied some blusher and a little lipstick and headed out the door. On my way to lunch I opened the sunroof to let the sunshine in, but now dark clouds filled my mind. I was shaken to the core and I knew it. My two conversations that morning had deeply unsettled me.

I felt like I was falling through the air at record speed, a horrible feeling that made me burst into tears. I admonished myself for feeling this way, but none of my self-talk was working today. To tell the truth, I was also concerned about my oncologist's warning from early in my diagnosis, urging me to pray that my tumor was estrogen receptive so I could take Tamoxifen to protect against breast cancer recurrence. I had declined her advice, saying I couldn't pray for that outcome because God was in charge of my being and only He knew what was right for me.

Then I remembered my oncologist's recent phone call, in which she said that the biopsies concluded my tumor was not estrogen receptive. I could tell she was disappointed and a bit concerned, since there was no drug to protect me in the years to come, but her words meant nothing to me at the time; I was still jubilant from my CCR outcome. Today, however, simple words from people I cared about shook my foundation as I assessed the doctor's message.

Uncharacteristically, I was filled with anxiety. The peace I once knew throughout this nightmare eluded me now. In desperation I looked into the blue skies above, crying out to my Heavenly Father, confessing how silly I was for feeling this way, especially after my miracle, but something about the recent words I had heard traumatized me. I prayed for an undeniable sign that would dispel my uncertainties, asking God for His peace to return to me, the peace that surpasses human understanding.

Finally I met George at a restaurant I had chosen because we hadn't been there in a while. I explained to him what had transpired that morning and reminded him of the oncologist's recent warning. George told me not to worry, reminding me to *stay in the day*, but I was shaken, feeling something I hadn't experienced since my diagnosis: fear! The more I spoke of it the more unnerved I became. I was heading into the future without a safety net!

I shared my prayer with George as he cupped his hands over mine, consoling me from across the table. He suggested this was the natural course of events after the trauma I had been through in the past months. He added, "Everyone has admired your courage and faith, even your doctors."

I held up my menu, pretending to look it over, continuing to pray silently, "Please, Lord, help me feel your peace once again." Then my attention drifted to the right of where I was sitting, and I couldn't believe what I was seeing: one of my favorite employees from a previous job,

Cheryl, was seated nearby, staring back at me in disbelief! I had never expected to see her again after she left the area many years before.

Recognizing each other, we stood up in amazement and screamed each other's names. She quickly ran toward me, giving me a bear hug as she whispered excitedly in my ear, "How have you been?" I answered as I normally would, "I'm good." In my excitement I momentarily forgot about breast cancer!

Still in her embrace, Cheryl sweetly kissed me on the cheek, as I began to correct my statement, "I should say, I'm doing well now. I've had breast cancer." At just the same moment the words "breast cancer" came out of my mouth, Cheryl gasped in astonishment, saying, "You've been healed!" They were words of wonderment. Drawing back from our embrace she looked shocked. I thought it was from seeing me after all these years and said, "So you've been in touch with people from our old office?" Bewildered, she replied, "No, I wouldn't know how to contact them after all this time." My mind whirled from her response.

"I'm confused, then. How did you know God gave me a miracle?"

She sighed deeply as tears slid down her face. Trying to compose herself she answered, "I had no idea you had breast cancer, but as you said those words God spoke to me and said, 'She's been healed.' I was astonished by the sound of His voice and simply repeated those words out loud. I didn't know what God was talking about until you told me."

Then she closed her eyes and placed her hand over her heart and shook her head reverently, deeply touched by the spiritual encounter. We knew the Divine had spoken to Cheryl; George and I witnessed it. Then she said, "I'm here today with my minister. I need to tell him what just happened. God has never spoken to me before, but today I heard Him loud and clear."

I watched as she scurried to her table, sharing her holy experience with her clergyman. She was still in an emotional and awestruck state when she returned and introduced him. I shared my story, disclosing that today was a particularly difficult day for me, being unnerved by some innocent remarks concerning my recovery. I told the pastor that for the first time since my diagnosis, fear and unrest had come over my spirit, and I begged God to put me back in His perfect peace, asking for His message to be undeniable.

After hearing my story the minister spoke, saying it was no coincidence I had chosen the very restaurant where Cheryl was also dining. He thanked me for sharing my story, saying I'd be in his prayers, reminding me to hold fast to the message God delivered.

Cheryl was God's messenger that day, and the peace of God flooded over me, once again enveloping me in His love. I was returned to His glorious presence, free from worry and fear.

. . . and so it was.

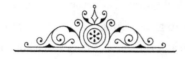

Meditation on Doubt

*Doubts are a normal part of life. We doubt things on Earth,
so it's easy to doubt things of God.*
Billy Graham

Planet Earth is a learning place, a place to grow our faith, abandon doubt, and move closer to God, becoming an example to those who want that for themselves as well. But if our lives were perfect and we had no doubts, how could we say we have a strong faith, when in reality our faith has never been tested? We grow stronger in faith and our bond with God intensifies when we experience adversity, allowing it to temper us in ways that only adversity can teach.

Sometimes we are afraid to doubt, afraid to examine our all-too-human feelings that perhaps our faith has been misplaced. We assume that doubt is offensive to God, that it signifies weakness and mistrust on our part. When this happens, as it occasionally will, we should look at doubt as a God-given opportunity, a stepping-stone to stronger faith. God can withstand any doubt we toss His way. He loves us enough to trust us in our grasping, imperfect search for Him.

Nor should we feel guilty about doubt, because doing so misses the point. God wants us to grow stronger in our walk of faith. A good way to do this is to look back at our lives, seeing situations that appeared hopeless at the time, no way out so to speak, yet somehow everything worked out. It is then we see that God was there all along, giving us renewed hope and promise. Looking back helps us move forward in faith.

At the beginning of my diagnosis, after the shockwave wore off, of course doubt wanted to invade my spirit, but I fought it with all my being, becoming even more steadfast in my faith. I did this by going to God in prayer and talking with Him as my best friend, pouring out my heart to Him, asking for His peace. *"And the peace of God, which passeth all understanding, shall keep your hearts and minds through Christ Jesus."* (Philippians 4:7)

I listened for God's voice and looked for His signs. I paid attention and He showed me the way, and I knew for certain that He would see me through the treacherous journey ahead. With doubt under control, we can face situations that appear hopeless with greater calm and courage. We see that God is right there with us, calming the stormy seas, our frail human ship navigating the rolling waves as we ride out the storm in the palm of God's hand!

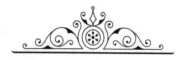

The Invitation

Nothing is impossible, the word itself says 'I'm possible'!
Audrey Hepburn

Many journeys include side trips, and mine was no exception. In the midst of my arduous journey, I had an unexpectedly pleasant experience. On a warm day in mid-July I fetched the mail and found, among the usual assortment of advertisements and bills, a creamy white envelope meticulously hand-written, a formal invitation addressed to me. The return address stated simply, "The White House." Inside was an invitation from Mrs. Clinton inviting me to attend the dedication of the Breast Cancer Research Semipostal Stamp, the first such stamp to be issued in U.S. history. Semipostal stamps raise money for charitable causes, and I was thrilled that breast cancer research would be the nation's first beneficiary of this effort.

The invitation was for Wednesday, July 29,1998, at 1:30 in the afternoon. Smiling, I shook my head in amazement, hearing myself say aloud, "Lord, so now I'm going to The White House!" My walk had taken me to unfamiliar places, but never did I think it would take me to 1600 Pennsylvania Avenue!

I immediately followed the instructions contained in the envelope to call the White House Social Secretary, accepting the invitation. She asked me to tell her a little about myself. I told her about the specialized protocol I was part of, including my remarkable outcome. She listened intently, saying it sounded like a great story, and wished me well. Shortly thereafter my phone rang again; it was a staff person in The White House calling back to ask if I would like to give a speech about breast cancer and the research protocol I was involved in. I remembered God's instructions, "You'll give hope and inspiration to countless other women who will follow in your footsteps." I accepted the invitation to speak, and complied with the request to fax a draft of my remarks as soon as I could.

While I was writing the draft, my phone rang once again, and I was told the First Lady felt that another survivor, Betsy Mullen, who had been instrumental in establishing the Breast Cancer Stamp, should make the keynote address. I of course wholeheartedly agreed and was thrilled to have even been considered. That weekend George took me shopping to choose the perfect dress for the celebration. It had been a long time since I'd gone anywhere in a dress.

On that special day I put on my new dress, applied a bit of makeup, styled my wig, and slipped on my heels. Looking in the mirror, I caught a glimpse of my old self, boosting my confidence.

I arrived at the White House and was seated. Mrs. Clinton welcomed everyone and then introduced Betsy Mullen, speaking about what she and other key people went through to get the Breast Cancer Stamp approved: it was certainly an amazing feat.

Mrs. Clinton also spoke eloquently about President Clinton's mother losing her battle to breast cancer and how important this stamp was to both her and the President. It was surreal being at The White House, listening to the speeches, feeling honored to be amongst the small audience awaiting the unveiling of this special stamp. Then a display version of the stamp was revealed; it was beautifully designed and received considerable applause and praise. Before leaving we were given gift bags filled with t-shirts and pins adorned with the stamp's colorful image. I asked for an extra one for my oncologist.

I knew this special day would live on in my memory forever, and I thanked God for whoever put my name on the invitation list (I never found out who), making me part of this historic moment. And I am proud to add that ongoing sales of the stamp have generated over $90 million for breast cancer research. The stamps remain available at the post office to this day.

Mine To Do

*Trust in the Lord with all your heart and lean not on
your own understanding; in all ways acknowledge him,
and he will make your paths straight.*
Proverbs 3:5–6

After a month of relative normality, the last thing I wanted to do was have more chemotherapy. But in late July, George and I headed for the Lombardi Center once again. After arriving, I was back in the saddle so to speak, and the routine was far too familiar! I had to admit, though, that I had missed seeing my doctor and the nurses during the past six weeks. They welcomed me back, and we caught up with the news of our summers. My oncologist wanted to hear all about my afternoon at the White House as I handed her the bag of mementos.

She then reviewed my latest lab results, noting that everything looked good, and finished the session by writing out my orders and a prescription for Cytoxan, sending me to Georgetown for my infusion. She also handed me the card of another doctor, a stem cell transplant specialist, who wanted to meet with me.

The thought of going through a stem cell transplant troubled me. I remembered my doctor in Boston telling me about the natural course of treatment for women with my stage of breast cancer, saying that patients who followed this regimen were alive and well ten years after treatment. I will always be grateful for meeting him at the beginning of my diagnosis, another angel pointing me in the right direction with a message of hope. However, I wanted to think that I wouldn't need stem cell transplant since I had had a CCR result.

George and I once again walked through the connecting halls toward Georgetown Hospital for my chemotherapy treatment. As we walked toward the elevators I admired the crucifixes on the walls, which gave me great comfort. Turning to George, I often said, "I truly believe that God walks the halls of Georgetown Hospital." I could feel it! I was placed in my usual private room while George went to get us lunch. By the time he returned I was already hooked up to my new chemo. While eating our lunch we talked over the subject of transplant, and I confessed I didn't want to go through any more treatment! But George counseled hearing what the specialist had to say—what would it hurt to do so?

The following week we were back at Georgetown to meet with the specialist; he was a tall, middle-aged man with a friendly demeanor. He welcomed us, congratulating me on the CCR. He asked me to tell him how I was diagnosed.

I told him my story, sharing God's communication and giving Him all glory, adding that God sent me to the Lombardi Center to receive my healing. I thought the doctor would now realize I didn't need the transplant. He responded that he was well aware of my phenomenal response; in fact, he knew quite a bit about me, divulging that he had been following my case.

Then he said, "Cathy, due to the size of your mass and because of its aggressive nature, even after having a CCR, no one can say for certain that at least one cancer cell didn't break free. A stem cell transplant could provide added insurance. At that point you will have taken every precaution to rid yourself of any stray cells."

Next he provided a technical overview of the procedure, which I listened to patiently. I thanked him for the information but explained that I would not need a stem cell transplant, as I knew I was healed. I explained that I would never second-guess God, nor would I need an insurance policy after what my Heavenly Father had already done for me.

I said, "Doctor, you seem like a nice man, and I know you're trying to help me, but as far as I'm concerned, I'm cancer-free and will remain that way."

He replied, "Cathy, I, too, am a man of God, and I hear and respect everything you're saying, but it's because you had a CCR that makes you so important. We've never done a transplant on a breast cancer patient who had a CCR. Your having a transplant would enable us to study you for years to come, furthering our research. Your clinical response was so great that we may learn things from you that will go on to help other women."

There were those words again, *help other women.* I knew all along God's plan was to use my body in conjunction with science to show the doctors how to do just that. And I was reassured that this particular doctor was a man of God and respected what God had done for me. With these spiritual issues headed in the right direction, I then raised the practical issue of how to pay for the transplant. Would my insurance cover it? This would be a very expensive treatment after my medical record showed an incredible clinical response.

The doctor agreed, saying approval could be a problem, but since my cancer was so aggressive, he would write letters of appeal if coverage was initially denied. In any case I would need extensive testing first—on my heart, my bone marrow, my blood, plus new CT and bone scans—to determine if I was a good candidate for transplant. Failure in any one of the tests could make the transplant team reconsider. Furthermore, the thoroughness of their testing could expose new medical problems that were in my future.

George and I thanked the doctor for his time, yet I was not convinced that I needed a transplant. During our discussion I was told I would have a compromised immune system for years to come; that definitely didn't sound good. The Doctor also advised that there was a certain window of opportunity to perform the transplant, after completing my final chemotherapy and before radiation, so time was of the essence. But if transplant was what God wanted, I knew I would go through with it. Only He knew what my future held, so I gave the doctor's staff permission to at least apply for the required testing, which insurance needed to approve before anything else could happen. In the meantime, I said I would wait on God for my final decision.

In saying goodbye, the doctor handed me a list of women who had already gone through transplant after a breast cancer diagnosis and who had volunteered to answer any questions from a patient's standpoint. Glancing at the pages, their names meant nothing to me at the time, and I slipped the papers into the transplant information packet I had been given.

As George and I left the hospital, I reiterated my opposition to going through further treatments. I was tired from six long months of being a patient, and I still had radiation ahead of me! I protested, "I will not have a transplant to give myself another means of assurance. I know what God has done for me and I accept my miracle." George heard the conviction in my voice, understanding what I was saying. As we rode along he patted me on the shoulder saying, "Honey, remember one day at a time. Give it to God in prayer as you've done all along. He'll show you the way." That was exactly what I planned to do!

The next morning I sat enjoying my morning tea at my picture window. I kept the house quiet on purpose; the purring of the refrigerator motor was all that was audible. I wanted to talk with my Heavenly Father without distractions, asking if a transplant was what He predestined. My prayer was for His guidance, knowing He would reveal His answer. I was serene as my prayer ended, opening my eyes to the beauty outdoors. I resolved to stay in faith.

One day, after some time had gone by, I went to the mailbox and found a letter from my insurance company, informing me that testing for my proposed transplant was denied! I was relieved! As I walked back to the house I said, "Is this your answer, Lord?" But just as I entered the house, the phone rang. It was George, calling to say that his company had just purchased a new health care plan and he wanted to give me the pertinent numbers.

I immediately contacted the transplant unit, asking if they too had received the denial. They had, but the doctor was writing to appeal the decision. I gave the staff member my new insurance information, and she said she would submit a new predetermination package right away. Some days later the staff member called back, saying she had sent the necessary papers, but each time she called to check on them, she was told the package hadn't arrived. She asked if I might try calling them myself, given the urgency of the situation.

That night I prayed again that God would let me know the path I was to take. The next morning I called the insurance company, but the phone rang and rang. I was ready to hang up when a woman with a kind voice finally answered. She explained she was a supervisor and didn't usually answer phones, but as she walked past an unmanned desk with the phone ringing, she impulsively answered it. I explained my story and said just to know that the predetermination package was received would put our minds to rest.

Something I said must have prompted a response from her as a woman. She took a deep breath and said, "This is what I'm going to do for you. I'm literally going to visit every underwriter's desk in the building to look for your package. I'll call you back at four o'clock sharp to let you know what I find." Clearly, the kindness I detected in her voice was real.

I stayed in prayer throughout the day, knowing God would give me the right answer. I felt I was being coaxed down a road I didn't want to take, but if it were clear that God wanted me to go down that road, I'd be his faithful servant and continue on. The phone rang at exactly 4:00, and the supervisor said, "Cathy, I'm happy to say I located your information." I thanked her for her persistence, saying, "That's just what I needed to know." But she continued, "I have good news, your insurance was approved."

Pleased, I answered, "Thank you so much. The transplant unit will be happy to know my testing is allowed." But she interjected, "Oh, not just your medical tests, your entire transplant was approved today!" Her answer took my breath away, creating a shockwave and epiphany all at once.

I quickly dialed Georgetown Hospital, giving them the green light to schedule my testing. The scheduling secretary was amazed that my entire transplant was already approved. She quickly filled my calendar with one test after another.

Looking out my window, I raised my outstretched hands toward the heavens, my gaze on the beautiful blue sky above. Through tear-filled eyes and a voice filled with praise I thanked my Heavenly Father for His guidance and faithfulness. I now knew irrefutably that transplant was mine to do.

A Mother's Prayer

Children are great imitators, so give them something great to imitate.
Anonymous

ummer was coming to an end but this year I wasn't just saying goodbye to Blake; Joanna was leaving for school, too. We decided to caravan out to Marshall University, our cars packed full, with the big dogs along for the ride. When we arrived, Merritt and his girlfriend, Karry, met us at Joanna's dormitory to help with the move-in. The girls had fun arranging things. They enjoyed a great connection, an older sister-type relationship, and their bond added to my joy and peace.

After a long weekend of settling Joanna in, it was time to get on the road. I envisioned this day when I was well, thinking how difficult it would be to let her go. But now, I wanted to shield my daughter from what was ahead of me, wanting her to enjoy her life again, to be young and carefree, far from chemotherapy!

Merritt hugged me tight, whispering in my ear, "Don't worry, Mom, I'll take good care of them." He was always my Rock of Gibraltar; I knew he'd keep his promise, smiling as I kissed him goodbye. Blake thanked me for a wonderful summer, saying I'd continue to be in his prayers. I hugged him tight, knowing I'd miss his companionship and spirituality. Next, Karry embraced me sweetly and said, "We'll all watch over her, Mom. You go and take care of yourself now."

For a few moments all the memories Joanna and I shared through-out her life came flooding back, our Saturday shopping sprees, mod-eling her new acquisitions for her Dad when we returned home. She was always my little buddy. We'd take our favorite magazines, snacks, soda, and the latest chick flick, get into my big bed, and enjoy our time together as girls. Every Christmas season I allowed her to take a few days off from school, her arm around my waist as we searched for the perfect gifts for everyone. While driving home we sang along with Mariah Carey's Christmas CD, enjoying our favorite selections all the way.

I could see her in my mind's eye when she turned sixteen. We gave her a new white car along with a white winter jacket and white Gucci sunglasses. She looked so pretty the next morning as she got into her car, looking up at me standing in the hall window, her face beaming, as she threw me a kiss and waved goodbye.

Then I thought of this past year, how bravely she saw me through months of chemotherapy, checking on me each day after school. Then I recalled the eight one-hundred dollar bills spread out like a fan on the kitchen table in June. She said the money was a gift to me, knowing my medicine was expensive and not entirely covered by insurance. I pro-tested, but she insisted, saying, "Mom, you've been so good to me my whole life, let me help you now."

My mind was filled with the memories of raising such a wonderful child. We were always proud of her; the years had simply flown by. It was time to say goodbye and leave her far from home. I closed my eyes and took a deep breath, determined to stay strong as I turned toward her and said, "Well, sweetie, it's time for you to enjoy your college years." She thanked us for all our help, and I hugged her tight and kissed her on her cheek.

George and I got in our car, the big dogs waiting for us. As we drove away the kids called out, "We love you guys." I threw them a kiss as I turned to capture one last glimpse of them standing together laughing and joking, caught up in a family reunion, complete now with their baby sister there with them. The siblings would continue their close bond throughout their college years, a beautiful sight to see, a true blessing.

As our car turned onto the highway, I silently prayed a Mother's prayer, "Dear Heavenly Father, please continue to bless my children and watch over them always." It was late by the time we got back to Virginia. I of course went straight to Joanna's room and turned on her light; it was obvious she was gone.

Many years earlier, when Joanna was a little girl, we bought her a package of glow in the dark planets and stars to stick on her ceiling. She and her brothers had a great time pasting them everywhere over her bed. During the day the planets and stars remained invisible, but at night they came out like the Milky Way. I recalled the many nights Joanna and I lay together on her bed, gazing at the light show as we talked and laughed.

Saddened, I turned off the light as I went to leave her room, and instantly the ceiling lit up. The planetary glow coaxed me back, and I took a moment to lie down on her bed and admire the ceiling's radiance. Somehow it made me feel close to her, spying her nickname Jo-Jo twinkling in the darkness.

"Oh, Dear Lord," I whispered aloud, "I'll deeply miss my baby girl, of that I'm sure!"

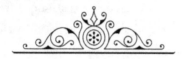

Preparing for Transplant

Friends are like rainbows . . .
they brighten your life after you've been through a storm.
Anonymous

The next day found George and me once again back to cancer reality at Georgetown Hospital. It seemed like I lived there, having one test after another, but in the end, all results were good and no other medical issues were discovered. I was now an official candidate for stem cell transplant.

One morning, while in prayer, I remembered the list of names the doctor had given me, women who offered to answer questions about transplant. I compiled questions in a notebook, such as, "How difficult was transplant to go through? Did you get sick? How long did it take to recover? Were there any complications? Ultimately, did you feel it was worth it?"

I began calling some of the women, and although they were helpful, I could tell transplant had been a challenge to go through, and they had put it behind them, not really wanting to relive it. I couldn't blame them. As pleasant as they were, I felt no hand of friendship extended.

Looking over the list, I came across a unique first name, Leda. On an impulse I called her, and she was warm and welcoming. Any question I had she answered fully, even personal ones. She was upbeat and encouraging, giving me the straight scoop with a dose of "you can do it!" I loved and admired the peace she exuded. She was two years younger than I was, a spiritual woman as well. The more I spoke to her, the more we realized how much we had in common. It turned out that she was even in the protocol, slightly ahead of me. On the long list of women's names, I stopped at Leda, knowing I didn't need to go any further. Since she was also in menopause due to chemotherapy, she encouraged me to call her late at night when neither of us could sleep. Over the months that followed we bonded; it was truly meant to be.

At my next meeting with the transplant team, the doctor introduced me to a nurse named Jane who was working on her doctorate. She had created a protocol to follow women going through stem cell transplant, knowing they usually developed stomatitis, or sores of the mouth. These sores were usually large, ulcerated, and quite painful. The Ph.D. candidate was trying to figure out what caused them, ultimately hoping to discover treatment and possible prevention. Her protocol involved taking daily swabs of the inside of a woman's mouth during and after transplant.

Her words rang true when she said she hoped her protocol would *help other women* in the future. I agreed to participate, although I heard myself say, "I know I won't get stomatitis, but you're welcome to study me." She looked perplexed, saying that, unfortunately, most women develop these sores. I replied, "God gave me a miracle. He wants me to have this transplant so science can continue to study me to help other women. If I don't get the sores, perhaps you'll be able to discover why I didn't get them?" She smiled at me, admiring my faith. Yet, I could see by the expression on her face she believed I'd still suffer the painful sores she observed. I signed the protocol permission papers and she said she'd be seeing me soon.

I was then given a date in October to have a special port surgically placed in my chest, with transplant likely to follow in early November. The doctors gave me more assignments: I needed a gynecological checkup to ensure I had no infections, plus a dental appointment for a deep cleaning to minimize the bacteria in my mouth. While I would be hospitalized, the doctors also wanted the vents in our house cleaned, making sure the air ducts were free of germs and mold.

While contemplating my three- to four-week stay in a small room in a secluded part of the hospital, I decided to compose a letter to family and friends, letting them know what lay ahead of me. I told them I would have my laptop to keep me connected to the outside world and gave them my e-mail address. After writing my letter, I needed the perfect paper to print it on, and at a local store I found stationery with a beautiful rainbow in its background. Rainbows had always played an important part in my childhood memories.

Upon finding the stationery, I reminisced about those happy summer days gone by. One minute I was basking in the rays of the warm sunshine, building sandcastles on the beach, when out of nowhere, the sun became obscured, the winds picked up, and the sky turned ominous. I knew it was time to head for the safety of home. The rain always began as tiny droplets pinging on my face as I madly dashed for shelter. I could see my mother standing on our front porch, beckoning me to run faster. Somehow I always made it to safety just before the torrents arrived.

Then, before the rain completely stopped, Mister Sun would peek his golden head out of the clouds once again. It was strange to see the rain and the sunshine at the same time, strange but magical. The winds would die down to a breeze, and suddenly the rain came to a halt. That's when the birds came out again, flying all about, as the world took on a fresh sense of peace, allowing me to go back outside, continuing my wondrous day of play. I jumped over puddles everywhere, and I looked up hopefully, yearning to catch God's magnificent masterpiece, the rainbow!

It didn't always happen, and in fact I would say it was a rarity where I lived near the beach, but when it did happen the rainbow brought with it many questions and a sense of wonder. I remembered calling out to my mother in excitement, "Come quick and see the rainbow!" My mother ventured out on our porch to experience God's artwork for herself.

Then I asked, "Mama, where does the rainbow come from?"

She reverently explained that the Earth was once covered by water, as man was not obeying God. She went on to say, "After the flood, God made a new covenant with man, vowing to never again flood the Earth, so the rainbow signifies God's promise to mankind."

"But where does it stop?"

"I don't know," my mother answered, "but they say there's a pot of gold at the rainbow's end."

"Who says that?!" I asked.

"It's an old Irish legend," she replied.

"Has anyone ever found the pot of gold?"

"Not to my knowledge," my mother answered sweetly.

My eyes followed the colorful arch down into the ground, somewhere far from where I was standing, making me wonder, where did the rainbow end? I never imagined I'd find the pot of gold in my lifetime, yet forty years later while undergoing cancer treatment, I'd find the real treasure at the end of the rainbow. This time the storm was not a summer squall, cooling a hot summer's day and creating a rainbow. Instead, this rainbow was chosen by me, with the rainbows of my childhood depicted on each page. I was preparing for three weeks of solitary confinement to have a stem cell transplant that would eradicate my immune system and place my very existence at risk. Yet God revealed to me it was mine to do.

I purchased the paper and hurried home to print my letter on each sheet, assuring everyone I'd be fine as I was in God's capable hands. Next and most important I asked for prayers for safe passage through the treacherous journey on which I was embarking. I printed about 300 letters, and included handwritten notes on many of them, realizing my busy life had kept me from keeping in touch with many of the people I was writing to.

As I addressed my beautiful rainbow letters, I came across a name I hadn't thought about for many years, my childhood friend, Tishie, the girl who went with me to the Billy Graham Crusades. Staring at her name, I wondered how we lost contact. We thought nothing would or could separate us, yet time had done just that. I decided to call the last number written in my address book, but a recording told me the number was disconnected. I wondered if I'd ever find her again.

When we had last spoken more than a decade before, she revealed she was a recovering alcoholic. She was divorced at the time, and now I didn't know if she had remarried and had a new last name, so I decided to write to her in care of her elderly mother's address, the last one I had for her. If the letter came back undeliverable, then maybe I'd lost contact with her for good. I didn't want to think about that, so on Tishie's letter I wrote a special note. The next day, as I mailed the letters out, hers was the last to go in the mail slot. I held onto it for a moment, praying that somehow she'd receive it and I'd hear back from her soon.

I never did find the leprechaun's pot of gold, but when I sent my rainbow letter to Tishie with its personal message to an address I wasn't even sure still existed, months later I would realize I'd found a different pot of gold at the rainbow's end—a God-given, golden friendship all but forgotten!

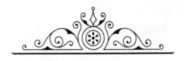

Seeds of Faith

Yea, though I walk through the valley of the shadow
of death, I will fear no evil: for thou art with me;
thy rod and thy staff they comfort me.
Psalm 23:4 (KJV)

*I*n October, Marshall University's football season was in full swing; we wanted to enjoy one last home game with our kids before transplant. We loved sitting in the stands cheering for our favorite team, yelling "We Are Marshall." But just before our trip, the transplant specialist called to say he needed to do a bone marrow aspiration on me. I'd heard it was an unpleasant test.

I asked my doctor if I could still travel the seven hours to the university once the test was completed. He said I could, if I felt comfortable enough to do so, saying the bandages would need proper care. As we drove to Georgetown Hospital, I prayed the test would be painless so I could make the trip to see our kids.

As I lay on my side during the aspiration, I focused on God, thanking Him for being with me. I can honestly say I felt no pain, and when the doctor said he was finished, I was the one most surprised, grateful I was pain-free, knowing God made it so. Rather quickly, George and I were on our way. Over the weekend at Marshall we laughed, talked, cheered, and simply enjoyed every moment of our time together.

Unfortunately, as with most good times, our reunion was over much too soon. Monday morning we were back at Georgetown to have a Hickman port inserted in my chest in preparation for transplant. This central venous catheter would be different from others I'd had, requiring daily meticulous care to avoid infection. George was given special instructions for tending it, and I knew from the excellent care he had already been providing that he could handle it.

Toward the end of October, I was admitted to the hospital and given an aggressive, heavy-duty chemotherapy cocktail that included my old friend Taxol. This chemo would kill any possible stray cancer cells in my body (along with many good ones), the first step in preparing for transplant. I prayed throughout the two days, drawing ever closer to God and my spirit.

The following day I was released to go home to cope with the effects of aggressive chemotherapy. The familiar bone pain, fever, chills, and loss of appetite returned, as my body worked to purge the toxicity that ran through my veins.

My blood count was followed closely. When healthy new blood cells reached the right level (and in theory, were cancer-free), I would be admitted to the hospital for apheresis, a process that harvests the stem cells for later use in the transplant. We were also waiting for fighter T-cells to be mobilized to help my immune system. On October 20, my blood count was satisfactory, and I returned to Georgetown Hospital. I have to say, there was nothing uncomfortable or difficult about the apheresis process. I simply sat connected to a machine (similar to the type used for dialysis) that filtered my blood for stem cells before returning the rest of the blood to my body. When the procedure was over a nurse showed me the bags of blood, telling me they'd be frozen until I needed them.

I was again released to go home, this time to await the call to be admitted for transplant. I didn't go into any of the dangers with my children that lay ahead of me because I didn't want them to worry. My mother asked if she could stay with me in my hospital room for the possible month long transplant. But I knew what I had to go through and I didn't want my mother or my children to have to sit there day after day, watching me.

The following week, my phone rang late one night; it was Leda wanting to know if I had any last-minute questions. How considerate of her, I thought; by this time we were close friends. Over the months I had learned that she, too, was a professional woman under much stress with her job. Although I hadn't met her in person, I loved everything about her, feeling as if I knew her all my life. We planned to meet in the near future once I was able, and she promised to keep in touch throughout my treatment. It's amazing how powerful women can be in helping other women!

As transplant neared, a calm washed over me. I feared nothing, knowing God would carry me through. It's wonderful how we learn to accept things, resigning ourselves to what lies ahead, once we're in harmony with the will of God. The call came in early November. My blood was nearly normal; admittance was close at hand. I reviewed my to-do list for holiday preparations, wanting to come home to a festive house after the transplant. The house was decorated and I had managed to get some baking done. It was nice to feel useful again, even though this Christmas would be small compared with our usual extravagant celebrations. All that mattered is that our family would be together again.

By mid-week I decided to enjoy a last bit of shopping before I entered the hospital. I thought about all the days of my life when even a day of shopping was taken for granted; today I was grateful simply to browse. While walking through a beautifully decorated store my mind went to God, praising Him for His faithfulness, thanking Him for all He'd done for me. I said I needed Him more than ever now, and I felt courage just to know I was doing what He wanted. Still, as the time grew closer to have my immune system intentionally destroyed, His presence meant everything to me. My talk was that of speaking to a loving earthly father, someone I could always count on, sharing that special bond from childhood.

Walking through the store, I continued talking with God, asking Him for his continued support and loving care for the journey ahead. In my prayer, I asked Him to send a message, giving me the confidence and reassurance I still needed. Finishing my request I came to an area of tall racks holding elegant greeting cards; lost in my thoughts, I accidentally side-swiped one of the stands with the shopping cart. A card that was sitting atop the stand slid off, and as it floated toward the floor I instinctively reached out, catching it with my fingertips.

Turning it over, I noted it was beautifully designed, depicting a large heart filled with roses. At the top of the card, gold letters spelled out the word *Miracles*. On the lower third was this verse:

The garden of life offers a thousand miracles,
and the promise of tomorrow is born of the seeds of faith we plant today.

This message took my breath away; I was awestruck. The card was blank inside, except for a smaller heart of roses, which might well have said, "Love from Your Heavenly Father." My eyes glazed over as emotion bubbled up inside me. I held the card for several minutes, reading and rereading its message, scouring the racks for a duplicate, only to find it was one of a kind! With this message meant for me from the Almighty, I was fortified and ready to go.

Later that day the phone rang; I was told to report to the hospital the following afternoon— transplant was now a reality. I was admitted to the transplant floor of Georgetown University Hospital on Friday the 13th of November, but I harbored no superstitions. I was firmly resolved to go where God wanted me to go.

The 10x10 room I would call home for the coming weeks was furnished with a hospital bed, dresser, desk, a couple of easy chairs, a TV, and a private bath. The window in my room looked out to another wing of the hospital, obscuring my view; still, it brought in the sunshine. George set up my computer for e-mail and we stocked the kitchenette across from my room with sparkling water and pink lemonade. The chemotherapy to destroy my immune system would begin at 11:00 p.m. sharp. Everything in good order, George said goodnight, giving me a kiss that would need to last for the length of my hospital stay.

Then a nurse came into my room and handed me instructions for keeping myself safe from germs: two showers daily using an antibacterial soap, washing thoroughly from the top of my bald head to my toes; frequent hand washing to the tune of "Row, Row, Row Your Boat" ten times; special mouthwash several times a day, in addition to cleaning my teeth with a soft, cloth-like brush that would prevent any small cuts. And, of course, I needed to wear a mask at all times while walking the halls of the isolation ward for exercise.

The long day was coming to a close as I changed into my hospital gown and got into bed. At about 10:30 p.m. a nurse checked my blood pressure; it appeared all systems were go, and she connected the big bags of chemo looming over my head to the catheter in my chest, saying she'd be back at 11:00 to open the drip.

For a few minutes I was alone in the room. The only light was on the wall above my head, giving the room a heavenly feel as I folded my hands and went to prayer. "Lord, I'm here to do your will. I know you are with me and I fear no evil. I believe you will take me safely and easily through this perilous passage, as I commit myself to your loving care." I closed my eyes, sighing contentedly and feeling God's presence.

As promised the nurse was back in my room promptly at 11:00, opening the drip to start the process. Over the next few days I slept a lot until George came for his visit, bringing me my mail and magazines to read. After four days of this intense chemotherapy, my immune system was gone. After two days of fluids and rest (and no visitors), I was ready to receive my own stem cells back into my body. I watched the nurse hook the once-frozen bags to the tower, preparing the life-giving fluid to drip slowly into my veins.

My doctors warned I'd start to have problems a few days after transplant. A day later, while on my walk, I threw up in a trashcan in the hallway; I was given medicine for nausea right away and told to take a shower immediately. The iodine soap ran in red lines down my body. I likened it to the blood of Jesus, feeling protected.

Day after day as the doctors made their rounds, I continued to improve. I looked through the window in my door, giving them thumbs up. I had told them from the start I'd make it through with ease, knowing God was with me. The days passed quickly, and I remained unscathed while facing Goliath, blessed by my walk of faith.

I was grateful to have my laptop with me. E-mails brought people's lives and the holidays into my room, keeping me company in a lonely space. I thought how kind these people were to keep in touch and cheer me on.

The protocol for mouth sores was going on simultaneously. Jane examined me regularly, but could find no stomatitis! On Thanksgiving morning when she came to do her regular oral exam, she noticed my rainbow letter lying on my desk and asked if she could read it. She took it to the window for light, and I watched as she read it to herself. I could see by her expression that she was touched by its content. She asked if she might take a copy to read at her in-laws' Thanksgiving table, where other family members were doctors. She said, "This letter says so much about your faith and what you've been through. The medical community deals with so much sickness, they need to hear your positive voice of faith in this letter." Before leaving she commented, "You said you wouldn't get stomatitis and you didn't. Amazing!" At the end of Thanksgiving Day, even though I hadn't been able to share it with my own family, I had much to be thankful for and recounted my many blessings.

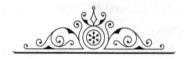

Freedom

If you think you can, you can. And if you think you can't, you're right.
Mary Kay Ash

On November 30, the doctors deemed transplant officially over for me. I had survived, persisted, and now I was being discharged late in the afternoon on my wedding anniversary. Although we wouldn't be going out, George didn't seem to mind as he entered my room to take his bride home. He held me tight and said, "Happy Anniversary, honey. Let's go home and celebrate." I said my goodbyes to the wonderful staff at Georgetown University Hospital. Their care and concern had been simply remarkable! George bundled me up against the cold, I put on my mask, and we headed for the car. As we drove out of the hospital's parking lot, George took my hand, squeezed it three times, and I squeezed back.

After a long ride in traffic we exited the highway just as it was getting dark. As we turned down our street I saw that our house was aglow with blinking and flashing Christmas lights. George had surprised me, making my homecoming all the more special. As we opened our front door, the big dogs lovingly circled me, competing for attention. The phone was filled with congratulatory messages for getting through transplant and wishing us a Happy Anniversary. Gifts and a card lay on the table. On our anniversary George always gave me roses, but this year fresh flowers were forbidden (as were fresh fruits and vegetables—too much risk of bacteria). None of that mattered in the least, though. I was home and the Christmas season was upon us.

George prepared a wonderful meal while we exchanged gifts, and then we turned in early after a busy day. It was so good to be home, where I could finally rest, and with George's assistance I'd rebuild my immune system. I lay there in his arms listening to him breathe deeply, feeling loved and safe. I went to prayer, thanking God for His goodness as heart-felt tears rolled down my face, having so much to be grateful for. I knew I'd awake in the morning to a new day. The odds had been stacked against me, but after almost a year of treatment I was still here and turning fifty tomorrow, Praise the Lord!

The next morning the phone woke us as my family called with Happy Birthday wishes. When my mother called she shared her latest Lucille Ball antics, making me laugh, and it felt good. My sweet Uncle Donnie called, too, saying he had a special message for me. He began ser-enading me with "Let Me Call You Sweetheart," a reference to the term of endearment my grandfather used for me when he called me "His ole sweetheart." That my uncle would remember this and bring my grandfa-ther's love to me on my special day was a wonderful surprise, and I have cherished this loving gesture ever since.

George brought in the mail, filled with cards. That evening, there was a birthday cake and another lovely dinner. I sat at the table in my pj's and bathrobe as we reminisced about our life together. My hairless body was shining from the shower I'd taken, when George looked over at me and said, "You know you're still the prettiest girl in school." I smiled at his sweet comment, thinking he was referring to when he was the football star and I was the cheerleader, telling him so. Then he replied, "I mean at fifty years old, you're still the prettiest girl in school and I'm the lucky guy who got you." He leaned in to give me a kiss, the kiss from way back when, when we were young, the kind of kiss you never want to end. Coming up for air he looked me in the eye and said, "I mean it, honey, you'll always be that girl to me. I love you."

I thanked him warmly, saying I loved him, too.

We'd been through a lot together: a war, a career in the Marines Corps, having babies and raising them, living in foreign countries, stressful work, and now cancer. I was so grateful for his love and devotion.

Just as we started to clean up for the evening, the dogs barked at a knock that came to our front door. We looked at each other, bewildered. Everyone knew I couldn't have visitors. George turned on the outside light, telling me to stay in the kitchen while he answered the door. I heard him speak softly, and then he brought in some packages. He beckoned me to my favorite chair by the picture window.

"Who are the packages from?" I asked.

"They're from Katy. She'll stay outside while you open them."

I heard a tap on the window, and there stood Katy, bundled against the cold December night. I was thrilled to see her and went right up to the glass. She spoke loudly so I could hear her.

"I've never missed your birthday in all these years and I didn't intend to start today. Happy fiftieth birthday, girlfriend. You're still older than me!" We burst into laughter, knowing that I am all of six months older than Katy.

I opened her heartfelt gifts and read the card, on which she had written how much she missed me. I looked up at the window, and seeing my rather wan reflection in the glass, realized I looked more pitiful than I felt.

I went up to the glass again to thank her for her thoughtfulness on such a cold night. Then she took off her glove and placed her right hand on the window; instinctively I placed mine over hers as we stared into each other's face. Naturally there was a sudden flood of heartfelt memories, being friends for many years.

She said, "I love you, baby, please take care of yourself."

I watched as she drove away into the darkness of a cold winter's night. Her gesture touched my heart.

After she left I found myself humming the old Dionne Warwick song, "That's What Friends Are For," as I smiled happily for having Katy in my life.

On a night I couldn't fall asleep, I decided to get up and make myself a cup of tea. Sitting at my kitchen table sipping the hot brew I turned on the television and surfed the channels. I was just about to turn it off when I came across the "700 Club." Pat Robertson and his co-host were just bowing their heads in prayer; I turned up the sound to listen.

At that exact moment Pat Robertson received a word of knowledge, saying a woman who just tuned in from the viewing audience had been healed of breast cancer. They praised God as I leaned forward in utter amazement, their words striking a chord, elevating my spirit. I knew God had once again orchestrated His communication to me.

I went off to bed, caught up in the spiritual moment, praying as I thanked my Heavenly Father for His perfect gift.

Christmas day arrived, and our family was together again, including my mother and Uncle Donnie, all of us under one roof. We were thankful for our many blessings and excited to start the festivities. However, I was still suffering the side effects of all the chemotherapy I had endured. The neuropathy in my hands and feet was unreal. Having little feeling in those areas, I had to make sure where I was stepping and to be careful of what I picked up. Thank goodness everyone was being extra helpful that day as I could be so easily worn out.

We exchanged gifts, and I was especially touched by the present my sister Nancy had sent: a beautiful music box that played "Somewhere Over The Rainbow," topped by the Wizard of Oz characters. Nancy knew it was my favorite song, as it was hers, too. We had talked about it years earlier, fascinated that two sisters shared the same favorite ballad. I fought back the emotions the song evoked, emotions based on memories of time spent with my beloved grandparents, reminding me of Sunday family dinners and watching classic movies.

Family and friends called throughout the day, wishing us a Merry Christmas. As we were making the final preparations for dinner, the phone rang once again. I answered with a breathless "hello" on its last ring. The moment the person on the other end spoke, I knew, shrieking in pure delight, that it was Tishie! My spirit soared. I thought I might never hear her voice again, but on Christmas Day she spoke my name and we exulted with excitement.

I retreated to my bedroom, wanting a little private time with her. She told me that the letter I sent to her, in care of her mother, almost didn't get delivered, but a dedicated postman recognized that the address needed to be updated and took a personal interest in delivering it. I told Tish of the prayers I had said over her letter, asking God to help her receive it. Tish asked her mother to open the letter and read it to her over the phone. They were shocked to hear the news about my health.

While we talked, I knew this little bit of time would never suffice, as we needed to put dinner on the table. I wrote down her phone number, determined not to lose contact with her again. We wished each other a

Merry Christmas, and just before saying our goodbyes she told me she would call me by mid-January.

Although she sounded great I was surprised when she said she was alone on Christmas. She didn't explain why, but I wondered if she were having challenges of her own. I returned to the kitchen, thinking of the odds against Tish receiving my rainbow letter. Praise God!

The family came to the table with Christmas music playing softly in the background, candles giving the room a spiritual glow as Christmas Spirit filled the air. I was overcome with gratitude, grateful to God above for seeing me through this difficult year. Breathing in the sacred moment, I reached out as we joined hands, looking at the faces of my loved ones as they bowed their heads in anticipation of the perfect prayer. I knew as I began to pray that God wouldn't disappoint them as words of love and appreciation flowed easily from my lips, thankful for our many blessings on this Holy Day.

Amen!

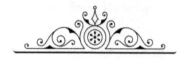

This Too Shall Pass

And we know that God causes everything to work together
for the good of those who love God and are called according
to His purpose for them.
Romans 8:28

As if the rigors of my treatments weren't enough to deal with, further adversity had been building in our lives since early fall. I had been without a paycheck for the year, and George's company now needed restructuring, necessitating a large pay cut for him. Between the loss of income, our normal bills, and the medical expenses insurance didn't cover, by late October we were coming to the end of our money. We sold our stock investments and used up our savings; we even took loans on our life insurance policies, but it wouldn't be enough. We fell behind on our bills, and debt collectors began to harass us. We realized that declaring bankruptcy was probably our only option.

Before I went in for transplant, we met with a bankruptcy attorney, who explained the process. He told us our credit would be destroyed for the next ten years! Hearing his words was like an out of body experience. I was nearly fifty years old and would be almost sixty before we could enjoy a good credit rating again; a decade feels very different at an older point in life compared with being twenty or thirty years old. The attorney further warned us that bankruptcy might not even be granted due to our higher than normal income before I became ill. In that case we would remain responsible for our debts, even though our income had plummeted through no fault of our own.

"Dear God, now it's bankruptcy?" I thought. But I knew I couldn't dwell on our financial woes as transplant loomed over my head; I needed to reserve all my energy and positive thinking for the ordeal in front of me. I reminded myself of the miracle I had been given, and I prayed that George would be given extra strength to deal with our financial difficulties as he helped me through transplant as well.

Any money we had anywhere, the lawyer warned, would be taken away. We might be able to hold on to our home due to my illness, but that was for the judge to decide. The future, if I really looked at it, just seemed to get bleaker and bleaker. I was even momentarily tempted to wonder how all of this could happen to George and me. But as we had done throughout this year of adversity, we decided to *stay in the day*, being grateful for all God had done for us. I knew in my heart God would take us through. I believed it, and held on to that thought for dear life! I told myself that one day soon, George and I would once again bask in the sun.

We had been given a court date for the end of December, and the attorney recommended strongly that I be there along with George, knowing that my presence would help emphasize the reason for our financial decline. I hadn't been able to promise anything until my doctor gave me the all clear after my post-transplant assessment, but my checkup went well, and the doctor approved my appearance in court as long as I took all precautions against exposure to germs. On December 29 I prepared to leave for my first real outing in a crowded place, the bankruptcy court.

George handed me the dressy soft hat he had given me for Christmas. I was unable to wear my wig during the healing process because even a small scratch from its netting could lead to a potentially deadly infection. My new hat wasn't a style I'd normally wear, but I knew it would protect my fragile head on this chilly December day. Then George zipped up my puffy jacket and wrapped a scarf around my neck as I pulled on my gloves. Lastly I put on my mask. I must have resembled a bandit version of the Pillsbury Doughboy. I turned toward my mother and uncle, who were still with us after Christmas, and gave them a blank stare. Childhood memories of being bundled up for the school bus came flooding back. We burst out laughing till our sides ached. It felt good to have such comic relief before we headed off to the courthouse.

Due to my severe neuropathy George helped me walk slowly into the lobby of the courthouse, where our lawyer awaited us. I excused myself to visit the restroom, and after washing my hands and replacing my gloves, I caught a glimpse of myself in the mirror. My skin was ashen, and I obviously didn't have any hair under my hat. I was a sight all right, but at least I was here, in all respects.

As we rode the escalator up to the courtroom, I could see people staring at me, the way people stare at someone with an affliction. I felt invisible behind my mask, but being stared at was still an odd, unsettling feeling, giving me greater empathy for anyone who lives with an attention-grabbing disability.

In the courtroom I looked around at the other people waiting their turn. Many of them appeared downtrodden, and I was saddened by their circumstances. My heart went out to them as I wondered what they, too, had gone through to end up here.

When it was our turn, George helped me navigate to the row in front of the judge. I sat there with my hat on, my coat zipped up, and my mask firmly in place. As the judge began reviewing our documents, my breathing picked up beneath the mask, making my face hot. Our lawyer leaned into the judge's bench with paperwork and my medical records. The judge turned toward me, taking in my appearance as our eyes met. I knew he was contemplating his verdict. As I watched him leaf through documents, our attorney's warning played in my head: "Judges don't like to grant bankruptcy to people who've been high wage earners."

Without realizing it my lips started moving, and I found myself in prayer as my heart beat faster. "Dear Heavenly Father, please help the judge rule in our favor." Over and over I pleaded for God's intervention. It seemed like eternity but it was really only minutes when the judge pounded his gavel, stating the bankruptcy for George and Cathy Davis was granted! I whispered to God, thanking Him for answered prayers.

George turned to help me get up. It was difficult for me to come to a standing position, never mind stepping out to walk. He led me out by holding my hands, walking backwards in the narrow area between our seats and the judge's bench; I could barely make it. The Judge was empathetic as I shuffled by, stopping in front of him momentarily, feeling compelled to offer my thanks. My voice cracking from all the stress, I said, "Thank you, your Honor." He remained solemn, nodding his head affirmatively.

George and I continued our slow pace into the hallway, where our lawyer was waiting for us. He looked relieved, saying, "Cathy, I'm glad you were able to be here today. I know this wasn't easy for you. The good news is that the judge is allowing you to keep your home. Other assets will be seized, however." We knew our family boat, for example, would no longer be ours to enjoy on summer weekends. Still, we had our home and we could start to rebuild our lives.

"Thank you, Lord," I whispered.

As we drove back home, George remarked, "Well, that went better than we expected, don't you think?"

"Yes, I'm glad it's over."

But in my heart I knew it wasn't really over. George and I were doing what we did best, supporting each other. We knew the true ramifications of this day; our credit was ruined for the next ten years. I had to admit I was exhausted from the mental and physical stress of the day. George told me to lay my head back and rest while he made some calls. I stared out my window as we drove along, thinking about all the years of working so hard and all that we had accomplished. Now we would have to start over.

Believe me, we had plenty to feel sorry about for ourselves. Yet, no matter how dismal the situation or how impossible things looked, how could I feel sad? God healed me of cancer, giving me a new directive in the process; my spirit lifted just thinking about my purpose. Seeing my reflection in the car's window, I smiled behind my mask, determined to stay the course, whispering, "Yes, Lord, this too shall pass!"

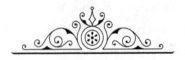

Smooth Sailing Ahead

It is good to have an end to journey toward;
but it is the journey that matters, in the end.
Ernest Hemmingway

 he following week, our phone rang late one day, and the
caller identified himself as a boat auctioneer. He was calling to say our boat was going up on the auction block over
the weekend. It was included in our bankruptcy. The man asked if we
wanted to come remove any personal items from it. I turned his offer
down and thanked him for his kindness, knowing it would be too difficult on George.

Every spring we spent our weekends preparing our boat for a summer
of cruising. I knew George wouldn't want to see our gorgeous boat one
last time, nor be reminded of all the money we had sunk into it.

Some weeks later, a man called and introduced himself as the person who purchased our boat at the auction. I felt a sinking feeling come over me.

He was elated with his find, asking if I wanted any of the personal affects that were still on board. Thanking him for his kind offer, I declined. He complimented me on the boat's pristine condition and the low hours on the engine. I knew he was curious about why we let this fine boat go. He seemed so genuine I decided to tell him my story. I told him about my aggressive cancer diagnosis and how God had healed me. Telling him that due to the loss of my job, coupled with my illness and medical bills, we could no longer afford the big boat.

At my story's end he took a deep breath, expressing how much he appreciated hearing about my miracle and what God had done for me. He then shared how he had always wanted a boat like ours, but a brand new one was definitely out of his reach. His family was thrilled about this boat. As he spoke, I remembered our own children's excitement when we purchased the boat brand new.

I told him I was blessed; my life was spared and that was worth much more than having a boat. I could tell by the tone of his voice, my story had touched his spirit. We chatted a bit more about what he did for a living, him saying he was in the produce business and asking what kinds of fruits I liked. He shared that business was good since people were more health conscious these days. I found myself encouraging him to enjoy the boat and make wonderful memories with his own family, content in knowing our dream was passed on to this kind man and his children. In closing he said, "She's a real beauty!"

"That she is!" I replied

A month or so later, there was a knock came at our door. I opened the door to find a deliveryman holding the largest fruit basket I've ever seen! Every fruit imaginable was piled high inside the enormous basket— whole pineapples, mangoes, oranges, strawberries, and cantaloupes. I opened the attached card. I smiled, seeing it was from the man who had bought our boat. He wrote to say that he and his family were spending weekends on her, making their own memories, adding that he so enjoyed my story and knew that one day it would encourage and inspire so many lives out there, just as it had inspired his.

I was finally finished with chemotherapy and looking forward to warmer weather. My kids were coming home for the summer. And I was so excited just thinking about it.

Merritt took a part-time job at one of the large, local banks in Huntington, West Virginia, while completing his degree at Marshall University. In short order, he became a respected member of the team—a successful loan officer— and received awards for his accomplishments. I was amazed he chose banking, as earlier in my career I was in banking as well. My background proved useful in running a successful company. Still, I urged him to consider medical sales for his future endeavors, being he was handsome, smart, and had a winning personality—a recipe for success in that field. But for now, he wanted to stay near his girlfriend, Karry, who was in dental hygiene school. And he also wanted to see the "kids" through their remaining college years.

As much as I would miss Merritt being home for the summer, having Blake and Joanna here was good for my soul. Blake was going to be a lifeguard once again at the place where the children loved him, nicknaming him Mr. B., and Joanna, who loved all sorts of makeup, acquired a job at Elizabeth Arden's Red Door as a makeup artist.

I knew that even with all we had gone through in these years as a family, I had set a good example for my children, one they would remember for the rest of their lives! When faced with a mountain, they needed to find a way over, around, or through it. My "way" was through my faith and trust in God. Whatever life brought them, they witnessed first-hand who to turn to in the difficult times of life.

Just as Proverbs 22:6 (ESV) says: "Train up a child in the way he should go: and when he is old, he will not depart from it."

As time went on my body continued to heal from the transplant, and I felt stronger with each new day.

On a picturesque day here in Virginia, I found myself driving home once again from my appointment at Lombardi Cancer Research Center. I was listening to my favorite music on the superb sound system in my car. I thought how lucky we were to have leased our vehicles, the bankruptcy unable to go after them, allowing us to keep our transportation. Still, from time to time, our lawyer's warning crept into my head: "Don't give your lease company a reason to check your credit. If they find out about your bankruptcy, they could take your cars away, considering you a risk." I couldn't help but wonder how we would ever get another car, especially since our leases were ending within the year. I quickly dismissed my fears, telling myself God was in control and that somehow it would all work out.

Deep in thought, I was startled when my integrated phone rang. It was George wanting to know how my check-up went. I told him my doctors found me in continued good health. I could almost see the smile on his face as he replied, "I knew that's what they would say."

Some weeks later, after George and I were asleep for hours, a booming racket suddenly awakened us. It sounded like a plane had just landed in our driveway. Our house shook from the thunderous noise. Alarmed, we sat up in bed. George looked toward me and yelled, "What the heck is going on?"

The next thing we heard was a banging at our front door. I turned on the light on my nightstand and looked at the clock, noting it was the middle of the night. The big dogs bounded up the stairs barking ferociously to protect us and our home.

George and I jumped out of bed, and as I slipped on my robe, the banging just got louder. "What in the world is going on?" George said aloud as he turned on the outside light.

I'm sure there was a look of alarm on my face, as that's how I felt inside. I shrugged my shoulders, puzzled as to who was behind our door.

George motioned for me to grab the dogs. I held them back by their collars, as he turned the doorknob at the insistence of the trespasser. There stood a large, bearded man in overalls, with a clipboard in his hand. George pushed the storm door open and asked loudly, in an agitated tone, "May I help you?"

The dogs were barking and snarling at the sight of the intruder in the middle of the night. The man spoke in a forceful voice, "May I speak with Cathy Davis?" My mind was whirling.

George answered, "What is this about?"

The man replied in a demanding tone: "I need to speak with her."

George answered sharply, "I'm her husband; you can speak to me."

Then the man beckoned George to join him outside. Before I could even protest, George was out the door. The noise outside was still resounding. I quickly closed the front door to cut down on the reverberation.

I stood there holding the dogs back and shaking from the intrusion. Just then George came back inside with the clipboard in his hand, and the large man stood there with the outdoor light beaming down on him. George made a gesture to the big man, indicating he needed a minute to speak to me behind closed doors. He then closed the door and turned to me, "Honey, the man outside is taking your car away."

I was in shock, disbelief; I didn't know what he was talking about.

Incredulous, I said, "He's taking my car away? What is going on? My keys are right here on the hall table."

George said, "Trust me, honey. He already has your car up on his tow truck; I just went outside to see it."

I was distraught when I answered, "Who is this man, and why is he trying to take my car away? We need to call the police and end this right away!"

George continued, "The man outside has been sent by your lease company to repossess your car."

I quickly responded, "Why?"

George replied, "The man explained that the tow companies aren't told the reasons why. They are just sent to take the cars away in the middle of the night when everyone is asleep." He then asked me, "Did you make the monthly payment?"

I answered definitively, "Yes, of course I did!"

George replied, "Honey, then there's nothing we can do about it tonight. The driver needs your signature, acknowledging you're aware the lease company authorized him to take possession of your car."

Instead, I went to our phone and dialed the automated line at our bank as I looked up the check number on the payment I made to the lease company. When the automated voice answered, I responded to all its prompts, putting in the number of the check I'd written for the month's payment. The automated voice repeated the check number and amount, including the day it was cashed. Proof they received the money!

The man outside was becoming impatient, banging on the door once again.

This time, I opened the front door and handed the man back his clipboard with the place for my signature left blank. I then asked the driver, "May I ask you who told you to take my car away?"

He answered, "Your lease company."

I explained that my payment was always on time, including the present month.

He said, "I'm sorry, ma'am. I have nothing to do with this. I just pick the cars up where they tell me to."

I said, "But there's been a terrible mistake here. Once I get this straightened out tomorrow, where will I go to pick up my car?"

The driver answered, "Ma'am, your car has already been sold to an auction house."

I gasped, feeling powerless and sick inside—all at the same time!

I begged the driver for my personal effects in my car, including my two-inch thick medical records from Lombardi Medical Center.

He replied, "I'm sorry, Ma'am, your car's been repossessed; you'll have to take it up with your lease company in the morning."

George tugged on my sleeve, urging me to let the man go on his way. The man glanced at the clipboard, and seeing I hadn't signed it, he handed me the blank copy of the form anyway: proof his company picked up my car. Bidding me goodnight, he turned to make his way back to his truck.

I stepped out onto our deck and saw my car tied down in the middle of the flat bed. The whole thing was shocking, unnerving. By now, all our neighbors' porch lights were on and dogs were barking everywhere, all having been awakened by the big, black monster truck.

The man shifted his growling gears as he headed back down my court, turning the corner onto the next street over, the engine resonating as he drove off into the distance. Suddenly, darkness fell over my property, and the night was still and quiet once again. I opened my door, stepped back into my house, and closed it behind me. Turning around, I leaned back against it. My arms fell to my sides as I pressed my hands against the cool steel of the door. Staring up at the ceiling, I said out loud, "Now, my car's gone, too!"

We had filed bankruptcy only a few months earlier, our credit destroyed. If I couldn't get this resolved tomorrow, what would we do? I then wondered if they were planning on taking George's leased car next. How would he get to work? My unanswered questions were beyond disturbing. My thoughts went to George, how much of this craziness could he take while still trying to make a living. He had his own pressures at his job, trying to keep the company going while making sure I stayed well. I told myself I had to stay strong, continuing to rely on God Almighty. While looking up at the ceiling, I prayed for God's help in the midst of this new problem. I was determined to pull myself together, for George's sake, as I walked back to our bedroom and climbed into bed.

I knew George was still awake as I moved close to him. Instinctively, he wrapped his arms around me asking, "Honey, are you okay?"

I answered, "I'm fine. I'm just troubled by the action the car company has taken. I'll never get back to sleep tonight, with all these problems racing through my head."

George reminded me softly, "Honey, stay in the day." He continued, "Throughout your diagnosis and treatment, we decided to stay in the day. That's what we do, remember?" I knew he was right. We stayed in the day, surrendering our problems to the Lord, and all that came against us worked out in the end.

George whispered, "I have you here in my arms, Cath, and that's all that really matters." The comfort of his words with his body pressed against mine lulled me to sleep.

The next morning, as I awakened I felt lost, knowing I would face an uphill battle.

Everything I thought of doing required a car. I thought to myself, "I'll meet George for lunch, and we'll talk this over . . . oh, that's right, I have no car!" A few minutes later, I'd think again, "I need to get some groceries for dinner." Again, I realized I couldn't; I have no car! Then, I thought about people who were really down and out, having no transportation at all, never mind the expensive cars I was accustomed to driving.

I decided to get up and call my bank manager to ask her to get me a copy—front and back—of my cashed check, knowing the lease company would need to see it. She said she would fax it to me shortly.

Determined to get this problem straightened out, I dialed the lease company. I explained my situation and was transferred from one department to another and getting nowhere fast! I was told they'd investigate where my car was taken, saying they would get back to me.

A few minutes later my phone rang. It was Merritt making his daily call from work.

"Hey, Mama, how are you doing today?"

I told him about my car being taken away, reminding him of our attorney's warning and expressing fear about his dad's car being next.

Merritt said little, but I could tell by the tone in his voice, he was disturbed over yet another problem swirling around his father and me.

Then he said, "I'll let you go, Mom. Keep me posted."

I needed to put my thinking cap on, to come up with a strategy to talk with someone who could help me. I decided to call the executive offices of the company. I sat down at my kitchen table and wrote out an outline of what to say, recording the dates of my payments etc.

I knew that no matter who made the decision to take my car away, the lease company would back him or her up, coming up with reasons to justify it. And once they pulled my credit report, they'd have all the ammunition they needed to support their actions. As I dialed the executive offices, I offered up my new circumstance to God, asking for His help in getting me through to the right person.

A receptionist answered the phone, and I explained my situation. I then asked to speak with someone who could hopefully turn things around for me. She was momentarily unaffected by my problem, ready to transfer me back to customer service, when I said, "I think you need to put me through to an executive, the decision to take my car away was done in error. I have just gone through a year and a half of severe treatments for aggressive breast cancer. My two-inch thick health folder from Georgetown Hospital was also in my car."

My words caused her to pause. She told me to hold, and she would transfer me to someone who might be able to help me. The longer I was on hold, the more I knew she was explaining my situation to someone. My lips were moving, but only a whisper could be heard as I asked my Heavenly Father to intervene.

A woman with a fancy corporate title answered this time, saying coldly, "Our offices do not deal with repossession."

I asked her to kindly hear me out. I explained I had paid my lease each month—faithfully. And I didn't understand why the company ordered the repossession.

She replied, "You missed this month's payment and after learning of your bankruptcy, someone in recovery got trigger happy, ordering your vehicle to be picked up."

Then, she said simply, "It happens."

I replied, "But that's what I've been trying to tell you. I made my payment."

She responded, "I'm looking at your payment history, Mrs. Davis, seeing you made timely payments each month, but this month's payment is missing."

I replied, "I'm actually holding a copy of my cancelled check for this month in my hand; my bank manager just faxed it to me."

She seemed surprised by my answer, asking, "Are you absolutely sure of this?"

I said, "Yes, I am."

She gave me her fax number and said, "Can you fax me a copy of your check showing the date it was cashed?"

I told her that I would take care of it right away.

She ended our conversation, saying she'd check on my car and call me in the morning. I thought to myself, God helped me get this far, I now had hope in tomorrow, and hope is everything!

The next morning the woman with the fancy title called back as promised, saying she received my fax, not knowing why the payment had not been posted.

I said, "Thank you for looking into this for me. I know you will make sure my account shows that it was paid. Now, we need to talk about how I will get my car back. I have medical follow-up appointments at Georgetown to go to. I desperately need my car."

She said, "Oh, unfortunately, I checked into your car's whereabouts, and your vehicle was already sold for auction. Once that happens, it's out of our hands."

Those were just the words I didn't want to hear. I was devastated by her explanation. And I knew she was finished with me now by how easily she said it all, obviously ready to end our conversation.

I thought to myself, what am I going to do without my car? And how will I ever get another one? There was no one to turn to. My family had already helped me in many ways during my illness, but I couldn't ask them for a car. I knew, too, that no bank could or would help me with a bankruptcy, and now repossession, on my credit file. While thinking it over, I realized there was no one out there who could help me—no one but God.

I prayed quietly for the right words, words that would awaken some sense of help from this executive. I tried to appeal to her sense of common decency.

"May I ask you something?

She answered, "Yes, go ahead."

"Can you imagine feeling totally healthy one day, being a successful businesswoman, and the next day, you are told you have a life threatening, aggressive breast cancer? I was on top of the world once just like you are now, but in one fell swoop, those words, breast cancer, changed everything for me. I lost my big job and everything that went with it. All the money my husband and I had worked so hard for over the years, went rather quickly to support us while I kept up with the intense protocol, which offered me a chance to live."

I continued, "And if that wasn't enough, I had a stem cell transplant, my immune system destroyed for years to come. In the end, we had no alternative but to file bankruptcy because not only did breast cancer affect me physically, it financially devastated us as well. Tens of thousands of women are brought to their knees each and every year with those four horrific words: You Have Breast Cancer. Can you imagine hearing those words and knowing what it will and can do to your way of life as you know it?"

Her voice lowered, "No, I can't imagine it."

I knew I was speaking up for every woman out there who did the right thing, created a good life for themselves and their families, and then, without warning, they were diagnosed with the insidious disease of breast cancer, stripping them of their health, their jobs, their financial wellbeing, their dignity, and more often than not, the loss of their breasts, as well.

She was kinder when she responded, "I understand you've been through a lot, Mrs. Davis. But your car is gone now so what would you like me to do?"

After being a loan officer earlier in my career, I knew the word repossession would remain on my credit report for some years to come. It would prevent me from getting a new car for a very long time.

I said, "I'm glad you now realize, with my cancelled check, that I paid my lease in a timely manner. I would like my credit report to demonstrate that."

She replied, "I'll make certain the word repossession doesn't go on your file." Assuring me a letter would be sent to the credit bureaus, stating my lease was satisfied as agreed upon. I told her I'd need a letter from her stating what she had told me.

I was on a roll when I continued, "There was obviously a mistake made in accounting to do with my lease payment. You now have proof of that. The error caused an unfortunate ripple effect. So I need something back in return after what has transpired. I would like to propose that I be reimbursed for part of my large down payment on the vehicle. To include the final lease payment I made at the time of my signing, along with this month's payment for a car that I can no longer use."

I let the words lie in the air as I prayed for God's intercession.

She hesitated and then answered, "Let me see what I can do for you, Mrs. Davis. I'll call you back as soon as I have some answers for you."

A short time later, the woman called me back, saying she looked at the whole situation, deciding to reimburse me as I had suggested. Never admitting they were at fault, but rather it was just some sort of "mix-up."

I thanked God for giving me the ability to think quickly and have the courage to speak up for my convictions. I believed He had gotten me to the right person.

After thanking her for all of her assistance, I reminded her that I still needed my personal belongings from my car.

She told me that normally people have to find their own transportation to the auction house to collect their belongings—if the car was still there—but she had advised the auction house to put a hold on my car. She then told me that she was sending a driver for me in the morning and that he would call me first. She wished me luck as we said our goodbyes.

Somehow, I felt good knowing I fought to protect my credit worthiness with a major car company and won. But no matter the victory, when it came right down to it, I was still without a car, and there was no easy answer in the foreseeable future.

George keeping his car was still a question. Would we hear the noise of the monster truck in our driveway in the middle of the night again?

I tried calming my fears, telling myself to stay in the day. I reminded myself that God was always ahead of me through all my trials, and this one would be no different.

This problem was too big for me to handle, yet they were small in comparison to Stage III Aggressive Breast Cancer.

Early the next morning, a gentleman called and introduced himself as Joe, saying he was in the area and was sent by the car company to pick me up and take me to my vehicle. I was up and dressed, so I told him to come along.

It was drizzling outside, so I went to grab my raincoat from the hall closet, but I couldn't find it. Instead, I grabbed an umbrella.

Looking out my hall window, I spied the man pulling up in my driveway. He met me outside his car as I walked toward him with my umbrella over my head. We spoke the simple pleasantries that strangers do, he seemed like a good ole country boy with a kind demeanor.

When we arrived at the auction house, Joe spoke to the man with the keys at the gated lot and beckoned for me to come along. The auctioneer opened up the lot, pointing to my car.

Joe told me to take my time. He would wait inside the auction house, and if I needed help to just toot my horn.

I had my own keys with me, and reaching in my purse, I pressed the fob on my keychain, opening the door. I got in. She started up like a dream, hardly a sound from the whisper-quiet engine. My favorite music started playing on my CD sound system.

I so enjoyed this car I thought to myself, remembering telling the salesman at the luxury dealership that if he ever got the model I liked in a champagne color, to give me a call. Weeks later, he called to say the car was on the lot in my chosen shade and telling me to come by and pick it up on my day off. I picked the car up in the morning, driving it all around town. I had owned several fabulous cars over the years, but this one was the perfect luxury vehicle.

After driving it all day long, I hated to give it up. I walked into the dealership, and they were already preparing the paperwork for my lease. Once I negotiated and signed everything, I got into my gorgeous new car and drove away. I called George to tell him about my new acquisition. He simply asked, "Are you happy with it honey?"

I answered, "Yes, I am."

He said, "Then that's all that matters; let's meet for dinner and celebrate!" The memories meant so much.

Back in the auction lot, the rain started coming down harder, reminding me to stay on task. As I opened my trunk, the box filled with my personal effects had tipped over. Spying my medical records, I placed them back inside. My raincoat was there, too. I slipped it on and pulled up the hood as I looked up at the ominous clouds.

Just then my CD player changed to Peabo Bryson, making me stop and remember happier times. I recalled seeing him in person years earlier. We were in the second row of the Music Theatre when Peabo left the stage to walk around and touch some of the people in the first few rows. He came up behind me and laid his hand on my shoulder as he continued singing his hit song, "Can You Stop The Rain" The audience went crazy and so did I!

Today the poignant love song touched me even more, as tears slid down my cheeks like the rain pouring down all around me. Standing there collecting my things, I realized my car was more than a means of transportation, it was an achievement I had worked hard for. But now, like everything else of material value, it was being taken away. We were being stripped of everything we had worked hard for all the years of our lives.

We had declared bankruptcy, lost our credit standing, all our money was gone, our valuable possessions were taken away, and now I had even lost my car!

The song on my CD player seemed to get louder, and as Peabo's voice sang out, my driver interrupted my disheartened thoughts, calling out from across the parking lot. "Do you need any help?"

I waved to him, shouting back that I was fine but needed a few more minutes. He yelled back, "Take your time, miss. I'm in no hurry."

I got back in my car, continuing to gather things to put in the box. Lifting my armrest, I found my Channel sunglasses case. Even my sunglasses were from a time gone by. I held the case in my hands and opened the box. The sunglasses were still in there, pretty as ever. I tucked them away in my purse, wiped away my tears, and collecting my other CDs, including Peabo's.

I got out of my car, pulling my box toward me from its place on the passengers seat, placing my purse on top.

The auctioneer saw me getting out of the car and hollered, "Lock her up, will yah, hon?" I nodded my head affirmatively. My thumb hit the lock button on the fob as I looked at my prize one last time, knowing tomorrow she'd be gone.

On the ride home, as the windshield wipers tried to keep up with the downpour, the elderly gentleman kept the conversation going, knowing full well that my car had been repossessed. Then he asked, "Did you ever own a boat, miss?"

I answered, "Yes, I did at one time."

He talked about his sailboat and how he wasn't able to use it of late due to all the storms.

I was lost in my own thoughts as I stared out the window. How much more could I lose? Better yet how much more embarrassment would we have to endure?

While I sat there feeling a little sorry for myself, the small voice that's in all of us, convicted me about my despondency, reminding me of my many blessings, one by one. What was I sad about anyway? I had been given a miracle!

God always had my best interest at heart; somehow He would make all of this mess work out for my good, Clinging to those words of hope and chastising myself for the pity party I was throwing, feeling silly for acting so dejected over a car, I vowed to believe in only good for my life.

Before long, we were pulling back into my empty driveway. I thanked the elderly gentleman for his help and kindness. He replied, saying he was happy to be of service to me.

I got out of his car and had started up my walkway when Joe opened his car door and called out to me. "Miss, I think you forgot your sunglasses." Looking down at my opened purse, I realized they must have slid out onto the floor. Joe walked up to meet me, placing the case on my box.

Then he looked up at the sky and said, "It's just like I was saying, miss, these storms are all gonna pass.

"Yep," he said, as he headed back to his car, "you wait and see. You'll be needin' those sunglasses before long. The weather's gonna clear up with smooth sailing ahead.

"Good luck to you, miss. You enjoy that sunshine, cause it's on its way."

I waved to him as he got back in his car and drove off. As I turned around, I smiled to myself, looking up at the sky as the rain fell gently on my face. I believed in a brighter future, knowing soon the sun would shine on every part of my life once again.

As I entered my house, I went straight to the laundry room, took my raincoat off, and hung it up to dry. I placed my box on the counter. Then I went to my answering machine, retrieving my messages. There was one phone call after another from my family, worried about the new dilemma in my life.

Merritt had called several times, asking me to call him when I arrived home. I didn't feel like going over all that had transpired, but I knew Merritt just wanted to make sure I was all right, so I dialed his number. When the receptionist answered, I asked to speak with him.

"May I tell him who's calling?"

I replied, "Yes, this is his mother."

She introduced herself, saying Merritt was such a wonderful young man, adding he was highly regarded at the bank by his peers and the customers. I thanked her for her kind words. She asked me to hold the line while she transferred me to Merritt's office. Her words touched my heart. Merritt was always highly respected no matter what stage of life he was in. I was always so proud to be his mother.

Lost in my thoughts, I asked God to bless him for always being concerned about me. Just then he answered, "Merritt Davis speaking, may I help you?"

I replied, "Hi, sweetie, how's your day going?" I tried to be uplifting to my children; they didn't need any more drama in their young lives.

He replied, "My day's going well, but it's your day I'm worried about, Mom."

I shared my small victory with the automobile company.

I was tired from the week's ordeal. I just wanted to rest and forget about the fact that I had no car, no means to go anywhere, including my doctor appointments in the city. And what about George's car?

Merritt said, "Mom, you sound tired." Telling him I was, he advised me to get some rest, and we'd talk later on.

The comfort of my bed called my name as the rain beat down on our roof. I took my shoes off, climbed into bed, and got cozy under the covers. I lay there thinking about all the things George and I had been through since my diagnosis. Each difficulty seeming insurmountable at the time, but looking back, everything had worked out. I could see the common thread as God took each problem and turned it into something good for us.

I closed my eyes as my mind went to Jeremiah 29 11–13, "For I know the plans I have for you declares the Lord. Plans to prosper you and not to harm you, plans to give you hope and a future. Then you will call upon me, and come and pray to me, and I will listen to you. You will seek me and find me when you seek me with all your heart."

God had a plan designed just for me. In time, it would come to fruition. How I handled adversities would be the stepping-stones to God's design for the rest of my life. One day, I would tell the story that God gave me to tell. The story would give hope to the hopeless and inspire countless others just as He intended. I would step out in faith to what He called me to do. As I drifted off to sleep, I prayed for God's continued help and favor in my life. I knew God was already at work in this new problem I was facing, even though I could not see the answer. I fell asleep resting always in the palm of His mighty hand.

I was in the midst of a lovely dream. George and I were vacationing somewhere beautiful, our troubles far behind us. Only the repeated ringing of my phone could arouse me from my sweet dream, as I had been asleep for hours according to my bedside clock.

I answered sleepily, "Hello."

Merritt spoke, "Did I wake you, Mom?"

I answered, "Yes, honey, but it's okay. I always like talking to my son."

The enthusiasm in his voice was evident when he said, "I didn't want to tell you earlier, Mom, until I was absolutely sure, but everything's been approved."

I sat up in my bed, sure he was talking about a new promotion, anticipating something wonderful for him.

"What is it, Merritt?" I questioned.

He continued, "Mom, I went to see the president of our bank today. He is a good man and very professional. I sat down across from him and we exchanged business small talk. He congratulated me on how far I have come in the bank since I first started. I thanked him for his kind words. He knew I had come to speak to him privately, so he asked what he could do for me. I shared with him all you have been going through with being diagnosed with Stage III aggressive breast cancer. I told him of all the financial difficulties you and Dad have faced in the aftermath of the disease. I told him that my dad is a retired USMC officer, and after a lifetime of doing everything right, you lost your car recently due to an error made at the automobile company. I mentioned that you are now concerned that Dad's car could also be taken away in the middle of the night since it is a leased vehicle.

"The president of my bank leaned forward and, without hesitation, he looked me in the eye and said, 'Your mother does not need any more worries while trying to heal from cancer.'"

Still half asleep I said, "I'm confused son; what's going on?"

Merritt replied, with excitement in his voice, "Mom, I went to see the president of my bank today to see if he could help us. The president is going to give you and Dad a car loan at a great rate. It's a done deal, Mom. You're all set. The president said, 'Merritt, let's make it happen!'"

Merritt continued, "Mom, this transaction will be like paying cash for a car. Whatever the total purchase price is on each vehicle you negotiate, I will then fax you the loan documents to be signed. In turn, my bank will wire the dealership the money. So Mom, go out tonight and pick out the cars of your choice, and work your magic negotiating them."

Touched and grateful, I held my composure, thanking Merritt over and over before we hung up. I couldn't help but think how my precious, little, blonde-haired boy—my little buddy, dear friend, and devoted son—was also such a wonderful man.

"God Bless my son" I said out loud in my room.

God had once again found a way to help us, this time through my son. I had to smile thinking of the Scripture, "With God all things are possible" (Matthew 19:26), and my spirit soared.

George's call came on the heels of Merritt's good news. The rain was starting to let up as George picked me up to look for our new cars. Negotiating with no trade and pre-approved credit is a great advantage, just like paying with cash.

George found an SUV that was already discounted with further rebates making it a sweet deal. I found a lovely new sedan with all the extras, but without the large price tag because it was the floor model; and I was able to get it for invoice.

We were thrilled when we picked up our new cars on Saturday morning. And after signing our paperwork, the finance officer remarked what a gloriously sunny day it was and recalling the terrible storms of late, adding it was a good day to open the sunroof.

George and I got into our new cars. As I reached in my purse to take out my sunglasses and put them on, I remembered how sad I was only days earlier about my old car, and today, I was liking my new car even more! I couldn't help but think about God's divine intervention, that our leases were coming to an end with no credit available to us, and a "mistake" was made at the auto company, causing a ripple effect, and putting things in motion, so our son could help save us before he went on to his true career in medical sales. Proving once again that God was always a step ahead of me in all my trials. All I had to do was surrender my problems to Him and believe!

Driving out of the dealership with George behind me, I opened my sunroof; the sun's beams enveloped me as I sailed over the roads. Instantly, I remembered old Joe's talk: "You'll see, miss, the sun's gonna shine again soon. You'll be needin' those sunglasses."

The old gentleman was right; God cleared my way, pushing another storm out to sea, and blessing me with "smooth sailing ahead!"

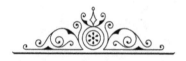

Section III
The Gift of Hope and Inspiration

My Message of Hope and Inspiration

Once you choose hope, anything's possible.
Christopher Reeve

*I*t's tempting to think that if life would only be calm and steady and throw very few challenges at us, we would be happier, healthier, and more content than we are now. This might be true superficially, but in attaining such a smooth-sailing life, we would also miss the opportunity that challenge provides us to learn more about ourselves and others. When life takes a sudden turn for the worse, hitting us hard with the unexpected, I believe it is how we come to know ourselves, how we cope and react to the unexpected, that has the power to either save our life or take it away.

A big part of our response to the unexpected involves analyzing what we can do about it. After receiving difficult news, it is human nature to inform ourselves about the issue and then to analyze and try to solve the problem on our own. If it's a problem we have some control over, we can apply various solutions and move on. However, it's when we don't have control over a situation that we can get ourselves into trouble by overanalyzing and believing in the illusion of control. We miss the real point of the challenge, which is that God has a plan and a purpose for each one of us, and He wants us to trust that the plan and the purpose are meant for our good, no matter how frightened or uncertain we might feel at times. We will grow in faith and love when we accept challenges as our path to self-knowledge.

God already knows the adversity we will face in this lifetime, and when we need Him, He will be there to comfort us and make our path straight:

Therefore I tell you, do not worry about your life, what you will eat or drink; or about your body, what you will wear. Is not life more than food, and the body more than clothes? Look at the birds of the air; they do not sow or reap or store away in barns, and yet your heavenly Father feeds them. Are you not much more valuable than they? (Matthew 6:25–26)

Many years ago, a year before my dad passed away, George and I went back home with our kids for a visit. Early one morning I heard my dad whistling in the kitchen, and fearful it would awaken my small children, I went to the kitchen to remind him we were sleeping nearby. But when I arrived there, my father was at the breakfast table, reading his bible and whistling happily, having been given another day to live and work after his terminal diagnosis a decade prior. He looked up, surprised but happy to see me, as 6:00 a.m. is not my best time of day! Still, the sight of him warmed my heart. Running my fingers through my hair, I sat down sleepily to join him.

I asked him about his bible, having given it to him some time ago. He told me that he read it faithfully every morning. I thought about how positive and courageous he was, never complaining or showing any sadness about his prognosis. He had a favorite bible verse that he often quoted to me: *This is the day the Lord has made; we will rejoice and be glad in it* (Psalm 118:24, NLT). My father loved to say it aloud, truly rejoicing in the day he was given, actually living the verse.

Not being totally awake I asked him a question that was running through my brain.

"Do you ever think about dying, Daddy?" There it was, out in the open, before I could take it back.

But my father answered me honestly and faithfully. He told me about the many sad faces of everyone he knew when he was originally diagnosed, especially while going through chemotherapy. He said that he could see the pity in their eyes, adding, "You know, the funny thing is that many of those same people who pitied me, died unexpectedly for various reasons: accident, heart attack, stroke, diabetes, or other causes. I have attended many funerals over these many years, while I'm still here enjoying life."

I said, "That's unbelievable."

My dad continued, "But the day the good Lord wants me, that's the day I'm going home, not one day sooner or one day later."

Then he smiled and said matter-of-factly, "You know, honey, no one is leaving planet Earth alive."

Wow, daddy had it all straight. After pulling on his jacket he kissed me goodbye, saying he would see me at dinner, as he whistled his way out the door, rejoicing in another new day.

We are all given a finite time to live and grow here on planet Earth. I especially love the words of Bil Keane, the great cartoonist: *Yesterday is history, tomorrow is a mystery, today is a gift of God, which is why we*

call it the present. We should remind ourselves to *stay in the day,* because truly, that's all we have, this day! If we use all our energy to worry about tomorrow, we have lost another day of our lives that we cannot ever get back. I have found this to be such a freeing way to live. Being present in the twenty-four hours of each day brings our lives into vibrant and meaningful focus, moments that are irreplaceable. And when we surrender our tomorrows to God, because He alone knows our future, we free ourselves most fully to honor the gift of daily life that God has bestowed on us.

In this final section of my book, before finishing my own story, I am going to introduce three special women whom God sent into my life at just the right moment. To my mind they perfectly exemplify *staying in the day,* as they learned to absorb the challenges that came their way with equanimity. They also taught me through their challenging lives that *hope and inspiration* reside on a two-way street. We may feel that our own stories have much hope and inspiration to offer others, but the fullness of hope and inspiration is best achieved through reciprocity. I gained as much or more from the women I offered hope to as they gained from me. Sharing my hope and inspiration with them became a learning process that surprised, humbled, and enriched me.

We will all experience struggles, hardship, sickness, pain, solace, acceptance, blessings and even miracles in our lifetime. And as we do so, hopefully we will come to appreciate that faith and hope are best defined as a means to cradle us on our ordained journey, whether that journey continues for a time on Earth, or whether God's directed path leads us to our heavenly abode. Faith and hope cannot guarantee us a more perfect or longer life on Earth, but they do allow us to live the lifetime God has given us, and to live it to the fullest.

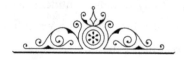

Leda

There are two ways of spreading light:
to be the candle or the mirror that reflects it.
Edith Wharton

oward the end of my stem cell transplant in 1998, something very special happened that brought new light into my life. One day, as the nurses were tending to me, a woman walked in behind them and waved. She was beautiful, with very short brown hair and eyes that shone, dressed in an off-white mohair sweater and long skirt, wearing the same color hosiery and shoes. Pearls adorned her neck and ears. My eyes followed her as she sat down without a word in the chair in my room.

The afternoon sun beamed through my window and fell on her as the filaments from her mohair suit shimmered, floating in the air. She offered me a heartfelt smile as the nurses continued their work; intrigued, I smiled back. As she sat there patiently, I have to say it surprised me that no one seemed to notice her but me.

The nurses finished and left. Resting my head on my pillow, I continued to stare at this lovely woman, confident she was an angel sent to keep me safe, at peace with this knowledge, when finally the angel spoke.

"Cathy, you know who I am, don't you?"

"I think so...."

At this point in my journey, I was so used to astonishing things happening that this ethereal visitor didn't seem at all unusual to me.

She spoke again and said, "It's good to see you and to know how well you're doing."

As she stood up in her ankle-length skirt, she seemed to float to my bedside, and I thought how happy I was to finally meet one of God's heavenly guides.

Then she said, "I had an appointment here, so I thought I'd come by to see you."

My angel had an appointment at the hospital?

"Cathy, it's me, Leda."

"Oh for Heaven's sakes," I said as I took her hand, thrilled to finally meet her in person.

She shared that her testing went well; the doctors were pleased with her progress. She certainly looked the picture of health. She, of course, knew all the nurses and doctors on the transplant floor, speaking to them before she entered my room. She sat down again to visit for a while. She spoke warmly, praising my progress with perfect words of encouragement. As Leda talked on and the sun's rays danced all around her, I knew she really was an angel sent to watch over me, and I whispered, thank you, Lord.

Even though Leda and I were in the same protocol, we might never have met if it weren't for transplant, as there were few opportunities to meet the other women involved. After leaving the hospital, it was wonderful to have a friend to discuss things with, especially when she said, "I know, I experienced that, too." On many of our late-night talks, Leda shared that in 1997, when she was only forty-seven years old, she had been diagnosed with inflammatory breast cancer. This type of cancer is highly aggressive and can be difficult to diagnose early because it grows so quickly. By the time it reaches stage III, when diagnosis is most common, it has already invaded surrounding tissue. Leda had been told that even after stem cell transplant she would be lucky to live eighteen months. Yet, she never complained or bemoaned her dismal diagnosis; instead she served as a model of positive thinking and can-do spirit. I cherished that in her.

It was in those late night talks that our relationship grew so quickly, where we bared our souls, and no subject was off limits. Mostly we talked about our faith and our reliance on the Almighty. Leda loved to hear my spiritual stories and although she never said so, I could tell she was in the midst of a period of immense spiritual growth, which was taking her to new heights. Our friendship was no accident, ordained by the Divine Himself. Yet here she was, more than a year after her diagnosis, healthy and strong, proving that negative predictions need not burden us while we stay in faith.

We celebrated our connection and did what all good friends do, met for lunch regularly, shopped, talked about our kids, etc. She also continued to make herself available to other women with questions or concerns, in particular about stem cell transplant. Somehow Leda always made time for everyone. She could make you feel like you were the most important person on her list. I could only imagine how she helped other women, too, who called fascinated by her lovely name, and were lucky enough to dial her number like me. You only needed a few minutes to speak with her, to be captivated by her warm, caring, and loving ways.

By early summer, Leda was thinking about going back to her big job in corporate America, as a Finance Manager for Bell Atlantic, to include philanthropic work for them, which involved travel to far off places. She had already worked for the company for almost three decades, but she was not ready to retire yet. She was doing so well that her decision to return to work concerned me. By now, I knew stress was a close friend to cancer. But even with Leda's grim diagnosis she vowed to *stay in the day*, wanting to live her life to the fullest with no boundaries. She was a real trouper. Shortly thereafter she rejoined the work force, filled with hope that the worst was behind her.

In November 2000, Leda was nearing her fiftieth birthday and I was planning a celebration for her with a mutual friend. On a glorious autumn day I set out to find just the right gift to make her special day even more memorable. Exploring a lovely boutique, I spied a sparkling crown to adorn her head, fit for a princess. I told the cashier that it was for a dear friend's special day, so she placed it in a lovely box and tied it up with a beautiful bow.

Leda returned from her latest trip and called to say that she was having problems with her breathing. She contacted Lombardi right away and they told her to come in. After her examination they gave her orders for days' worth of testing.

She called nightly to tell me of the doctor's suspicions. They were concerned her problems were related to congestive heart failure due to all the chemotherapy she endured. After her testing was complete, she was given an appointment to come to Lombardi and discuss her problem. She promised to call me when she had some answers. I waited and prayed, but her call never came. Instead, a few days later, she e-mailed me with the bad news. In the course of investigating her symptoms, the doctors discovered that her cancer had spread, this time to her lungs.

With all she was going through, we didn't get together for her fiftieth birthday, so I took her wrapped present and placed it on the upper shelf of my closet. I told myself that I would give it to her next year instead.

At this point Leda and her husband had some hard decisions to make about their future. Although they had deep roots in our region, they decided to retire and move to Myrtle Beach, S.C., where they loved the ocean and golf and would also be close to Leda's daughter and grandson, Graham. I can't think of a more comforting or life-affirming way to live out one's days. We were also grateful that Leda's oncologist, who had seen her through so much, was moving to Duke University Hospital in North Carolina, close enough that Leda could travel up for ongoing care. Her new environs would give her the support she needed in all possible ways. She would be missed, but at the same time I was happy for her, too!

Leda loved Christmas as much as I did. She planned to move in January, but even with all she was going through, she was determined to make this a memorable Christmas and joined her daughter and family in Atlanta. January came way too fast and with it my dear friend moved to South Carolina. We vowed to stay in touch and to make trips to get together. We kept our promise through regular e-mails and phone calls.

In October 2001, while I was preparing to have my annual post-protocol checkup, I sent an e-mail to all my family and friends about my yearly testing, assuring them that I was fine but that their prayers would be greatly appreciated. Ever so thoughtful, Leda called and of course she cheered me on. Later that night she followed up with her reply, saying she knew I would stay healthy, because Jesus had plans for me. Guided by her deep compassion for others, she told me this with great joy even as her own disease worsened.

I was hoping to travel to see her for her birthday that year, but sadly, her health worsened and she was hospitalized on her fifty-first birthday. It quickly became apparent that she was losing her life to breast cancer. Yet, she had outlived the discouraging prediction first given to her in 1997. Now it was time for Leda to go home. When the call came in from her daughter, Stacy, that she was gone, I was devastated.

I must confess that when I first set out to organize this book, I thought about my beautiful friend Leda. I was troubled that her story did not seem to offer complete hope to other women, given that she did not survive her ordeal. At the time, I even considered leaving Leda out of my story, wanting to convey a consistent message of hope, free from discouragement. How could including Leda accomplish that? Isn't death the ultimate discouragement?

However, in thinking it through, I realized that Leda's story was part of a journey, not an either/or experience that either contains hope or it doesn't. Instead, I realized that Leda represented genuine hope of its own kind. In her case, she maintained hope for surviving longer than predicted, to dance at her son's wedding, watch a beloved daughter and grandchild thrive, and enjoy a well-deserved retirement, spending time with her husband and family. Despite her health issues she made the effort to relocate, set up a new household, engage her community, play golf, swim, and simply enjoy every single moment of life she could muster. And through it all she never griped or protested—instead she remained cheerful and encouraging. If that is not hope, I don't know what is.

We had been on this journey partly together, and she had taught me so much and offered so much support and love that I was suddenly ashamed of ever thinking I shouldn't include her in my book. Leda, forgive me. Through your example you taught me to see hope in all its depth and splendor.

Many years later, while reorganizing my closet, I spied the wrapped birthday gift that I was never able to give Leda. I was momentarily saddened by the thought. Yet after all this time, I suddenly realized that the crown I chose for her birthday was merely a symbol of the true crown she received. Yes, Leda received a crown all right, but not a bejeweled one. Instead, I knew she had received the Crown of Life, earned the real way, through abiding faith and staying strong through the trials of life, facing each day with hope, love, fortitude, courage, and character. On the day she died, no longer bound by a body in pain, God's angels rejoiced at the example she set here on Earth. And with the gates of heaven open wide, they welcomed her back home for all time.

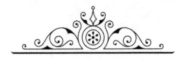

Tish

If you find it in your heart to care for somebody else,
you will have succeeded.
Maya Angelou

t's amazing to contemplate God's plan for us, no matter our circumstance in the now. God's plan may be in the next step we take, or an unexpected turn we make. And yet we have no prior knowledge of His plan, until one day it just shows up, and even then we may not recognize it for what it is, until sufficient time has elapsed.

Tish's story is a shining example of how God works in our lives, taking us safely through anything, even seemingly insurmountable obstacles. When we trust the outcome as part of His Divine plan, God takes us on a new journey, lifting us higher than we ever dreamed possible!

At the time Tish and I reconnected, after so many decades apart and at the very moment I was emerging from the rigors of cancer treatment, I was happy just to know that we were back in touch. I had no idea at the time what God was planning for the two of us, nor could I have imagined it with all that was going on in my life.

But when my mother returned home to Massachusetts, after her stay with us over the Christmas holidays, she was once again instrumental in guiding me towards God's master plan. She called me on New Year's Eve, 1998, to say that she had run into Tish's sister at the nearby mall, not having seen her in many years. My mother told her that Tish and I had talked on Christmas Day and how excited we were to find each other again. Then my mother asked how Tish was really doing? Her sister disclosed that she was living alone in a one-room apartment outside of Boston. She seemed troubled when she confessed that Tish was abusing alcohol again and the family now feared for her very existence.

I could hear in my mother's voice the sadness she felt for the way Tish was living. We reminisced about old times, all the fun and laughter Tish and I shared in our younger years. Then my mother asked, "Isn't there any way you could help her?" Rephrasing her question she said, "Maybe you could help each other? By finding her the help she needs and then bringing her to Virginia? She could help you as you continue to recover yourself."

I was surprised by her question. "How could I help Tish, at this late date?"

"You say God wants you to help other women. What better way to start than to help your childhood friend?"

My mother's words ignited my spirit. Yet, I pondered her question, thinking that although there was nothing I wouldn't do to help Tish, this seemed an impossible task. She lived outside Boston and I lived in Virginia. We hadn't seen each other in almost a quarter century. I'd just gone through transplant, radiation still lay ahead of me, and now George's job was shaky.

But my mother pushed on. "Just think, Tish could accompany you to your radiation treatments as she heals from alcoholism." She made it sound so simple, yet at the same time wonderful! I told my mother I'd think about it, but I highly doubted Tish would just pack up and move to Virginia.

In closing she said, "Maybe it's yours to do, Cathy. Think about it."

Putting the wheels in motion, I went downstairs and looked at my guest bedroom and bath. Standing there looking at this unused space, I knew it could be a perfect place for Tish to live and heal. My mother's suggestion kept running through my head, but there were still so many unanswered questions. Would Tish even admit to abusing alcohol? Did she have proper insurance to seek treatment before coming to my home? Would she even want treatment? What about her job, her apartment, her friends, possibly even her grown children, having to give it all up to come live with me?

When George arrived home, I told him about my mother's talk. He responded, as I knew he would: "Honey, would helping Tish make you happy?" Answering from my heart I said, "Yes, I think it would make me very happy to help my old friend."

As George and I continued our talk about Tish, I explained that if we moved forward, it would be a long-term commitment on our part. He warned, "Honey, I know you're excited, but there's something I want you to hear. Tish has been through a lot during these years of alcoholism, and although she may sound the same, she's not the same old friend you once knew. During these decades apart your lives have taken you down different roads, and the disease has changed her in ways you'll never understand. As long as you remember that, if she accepts your offer it could work."

I knew what he was trying to say. I would remember his words as I continued to pray about the possibility of my offer.

By the middle of January, after my children returned to school and after the decorations were put away, I still hadn't heard back from Tish as she had promised. Days went by with no word so I began calling her. Her phone rang and rang, with no answering machine to leave a message. I prayed for her nightly, asking for guidance and wondering how I could help her.

Each time I told my mother that I was getting nowhere fast, she continued to urge me to keep trying, saying, "Cathy, you could be the one to save her life. Maybe it's God's plan for the two of you?" The very next day I passed by a church sign that seemed to speak to me. Spelled out in capital letters was *PERSEVERANCE*. It became my mantra.

And so my quest of hope continued, when finally, one evening, on the fourth ring Tish finally answered, saying she had just come in from work. I was elated to hear her voice again. We settled into a long conversation and talked for hours, sharing our lives. I told her about God speaking to me while I was in Boston and that I knew, right then and there, that I would be given a miracle. She wasn't surprised as we continued to talk about our spiritual lives and reminisced about our youth, recalling our close walk with God. We talked about our many sleepovers, lying in her big bed, staring up at the stars, wondering what God had in store for us.

As we continued to talk, I felt prompted to ask the hard question: was she really suffering from alcoholism, or was her family perhaps exaggerating?

She answered by telling me about the many rehabilitation facilities she'd been in over the years, trying desperately to get the "monkey off her back." But time and time again, after returning to her old life with all its problems, no matter how hard she tried, ultimately she found herself back in the same mess, picking up a drink. She described her life living in her efficiency in a bad part of town; it was all she could afford, saying it was within walking distance of her job. She said her children lived in the South, and they hadn't seen her healthy in a long time. She had no real support system.

"God bless her," I said to myself. She had been honest with me, knowing I wouldn't judge her, but I was sick inside hearing all she'd gone through.

As she continued, it didn't surprise me when she told me that she worked in sales at a small retail store, as she had a winning personality and was always good at working with people. The bright spot was that she made it to work every day without fail. She didn't think her coworkers knew she was an alcoholic.

My mother's voice came back to me: "Why not make Tishie the first woman you help?" I knew she was thirsting for hope, and that obtaining the help she urgently needed and finding a place to heal and be loved could and would give her that hope. I felt the spirit of God urging me on, so I asked, "Tishie, would you like to get well?"

She answered, "Of course I would." I smiled at those four simple words that would change everything.

I offered to help Tish enter a detox facility near Boston, knowing that professional help would give her the best chance for beginning the road to recovery. Once she completed treatment, we would be thrilled to have her come live with us in Virginia to continue healing for as long as she needed us. When I asked her how that sounded to her, she sighed, trying to keep her emotions in check, and said, "Oh my goodness, it sounds too good to be true."

Since I had called her just as she came in from work, I told her I'd call back later that evening after she'd had a chance to digest my proposal. Not wanting her to feel pressured, I added, "Whatever your decision, Tishie, I'm just glad we're back in touch."

She said, "I am, too," ending our conversation with a heartfelt, "I love you, Cath."

"I love you, too, Tish."

I went to tell George that I finally reached Tishie. He laughed, saying, "I figured that out, Honey. You've been talking and laughing for hours." He could easily see my excitement; I knew he was happy for me, having something else to concentrate on other than cancer treatments!

Next I called my mother, telling her it was all in God's hands now. I knew that if this were His plan, Tish would move to Virginia; otherwise He'd help her in another way.

When I called Tish back later that evening, she picked up on the first ring. She shared with me that she had called her mother to discuss my offer, and her mom thought it was a great idea. Then I asked, "What do *you* think about it?" I was prepared to hear that the prospect of changing her life so drastically would be too much for her to handle. It would be a huge leap of faith for anyone, never mind someone with all that Tish had going on.

Instead she said, "I'd like to come to Virginia to heal and live with you." I was touched and shocked at the same time, and asked, "When do you want to make the move?" She answered, "As soon as possible!"

We hadn't seen each other in nearly 25 years, and if God hadn't guided my rainbow letter to her, I might never have found her again. Yet tonight Tishie accepted my offer to come live with me, giving us both time to heal from the afflictions we suffered. I was overcome with gratitude to God.

In closing I told her that I would get busy finding her a detox facility nearby. She had sounded so normal throughout our conversation that I was compelled to ask one final question: "Tishie, have you been drinking tonight?"

She answered candidly, "That's what I do, Cath. I'm an alcoholic!"

That night I thought about all that Tish would have to go through to move: being admitted to a hospital, going through the agony of detox, then attending all-day classes on recovery. She would be hospitalized for three to four weeks. Assuming all went well to that point, she would be released to start her new life. But she would no longer have a job, she had no savings, and she couldn't drive because she had lost her license due to drinking. She would move to a place she'd never been, where she knew exactly two people (George and me), and where the future was really just a giant question mark. All she had were promises from someone she hadn't laid eyes on since we were in our twenties!

When my alarm rang the next morning, I awoke with a renewed sense of purpose; I had a job to do. I began by tracking down Tish's health insurance benefits and then locating an appropriate detox/rehab program for her. This effort required many phone calls and a few dead ends, as people I spoke with were more or less helpful. But perseverance always wins, and it turned out that the best program for Tish was located at a hospital just a few miles from her front door. God's master plan had positioned her perfectly for the intervention!

Ironically, though, the director of the detox/rehab program told me that Tish would have to present herself in an inebriated state in order to be considered for admission. That meant she would need someone with her to ensure that she arrived safely, so I asked Tish for the name of a friend who might be able to help locally. She gave me the name and number of a woman from work.

When I spoke with this woman, she was shocked to learn that Tish was an alcoholic. She said, "I work with her several days a week, and she's been to my home for dinner, but I've never seen her drink. Are you sure she's an alcoholic?" It amazed me that Tish was able to hide her reality from the people who surrounded her. It saddened me to think how much physical and emotional energy it must take to live this way, and how the diversion of so much energy drains one's potential for a healthy life. I told the friend that Tish was in a dire state.

Her friend wanted to help, so we arranged for her to take Tish to the hospital the following Monday at 6 a.m. She would be Tish's advocate and do everything in her power to help her be admitted.

We now had everything in place for Tish to begin her journey into healing. On Sunday night I called her, and she said her small room was cleaned out and she was ready to close the door on her old life. She had only one remaining night to get through before her admission into hope! We both knew she had challenging times ahead, but from the enthusiasm in her voice I believed she was ready.

We were excited to think we'd finally see each other face to face in a few weeks. I reminded her to drink up that night, an odd request on my part, but we understood the requirement. Before we hung up I reminded her that I was there for her all the way, and she answered sweetly, "I know you are."

I prayed all night long and into Monday morning as I stared outside at the cold February day, asking for God's intervention. Finally, I received a call from Tish's friend, who said, "She was in rough shape this morning, but after a thorough examination, she was admitted." Mission accomplished! I thanked her for her kindness and promised to keep her posted on Tish's recovery.

Just before dinner that evening I received a call from Tish's doctor. He said she was in detox, wanting treatment and needing it badly. He also said she was severely malnourished, which I hadn't thought to visualize during our phone calls, but of course it must be so, given the ravages of alcoholism. The doctor said Tish would attend rehabilitation classes when she was stronger. He asked if it were true that Tish would eventually come to live with me. I told him that was correct. He wanted to make sure I understood what a huge commitment this would be. Then he asked when I had seen her last. When I replied it was almost a quarter of a century the air went dead; he was lost for words. I assured him our bond from childhood was strong and that I was recovering also, not from alcoholism but from breast cancer. We would be helping each other.

Days passed by. Each morning I sat at my front window and prayed. From what I knew about detox, Tish was going through hell right now. I asked God for safe passage through this difficult time. A few days after hearing from the doctor that Tish was weathering the detox as well as she could, Tish was able to call me herself. She was now attending classes daily, learning new things about herself and how to handle alcohol in any situation. She sounded physically weak but determined.

The day finally arrived when the doctor said Tish was ready for discharge. He called to say that she still had a lot of healing to do, both physically and mentally. She would have ups and downs for some time to come and cautioned me not to give up on her during the down times. I knew that was my chief job: to keep hope alive.

We set out on the drive north in George's sturdy Suburban, making careful but steady progress through the wintry fare of snow and ice. I could hardly contain myself as we pulled into the hospital's parking lot, putting on my hat to protect myself from the bitter cold outside. In my excitement as we entered the crowded reception area, I walked right past Tish; George recognized her and called me back. I ran to her, squealing with excitement as we embraced and looked into each other's faces. Her battle with alcohol had taken its toll. She was frighteningly thin and her eyes were sunken. Her thick chestnut hair was wild, needing a trim. But to me she was a beautiful sight.

She was wearing faded jeans and a well-worn navy fleece zip-up jacket. George asked about her luggage but she said she had none, not even a winter coat to wear. She stood there clutching a battered shopping bag containing only a few mementoes. I could see that hope had its work cut out for it.

After our long ride back home and a good night's sleep, Tish quickly came to relish her new life in Virginia, declaring that her room in our house was a palace compared to her former space. During the first few days, she settled in, slept late, and ate well. I peeked in on her each morning, amazed that after all these years we were back together again. I knew it was by God's design and I was content to let Him lead the way!

We soon created a household rhythm. Tish focused on regaining her health, which I encouraged in all ways from a good diet to plenty of rest and recreation. She also accompanied me to radiation, the last step of the protocol, providing support and companionship, doing her part to help me. Afterwards we would go out for lunch, sharing a sandwich and good conversation.

Yet as time progressed I could easily see she was experiencing the ups and downs her doctor predicted. She struggled with anxiety and depression, to the point of needing medication, but the rehab program had released her without any. Without a job or insurance now, she was in a bind, so I called our family practitioner, a caring man, and asked if he could help.

He said to come in right away, and after examining Tish he couldn't believe she hadn't been given medication before leaving rehab, saying it was a recipe for disaster and a miracle that she hadn't relapsed. I sat there unable to imagine all that she'd been through in the lost years, but I knew the hand of God was upon her. We left the doctor's office with a bag full of samples and a feeling of peace.

After some time passed, Tish began to feel that she should look for a job, not wanting us to pay for everything she needed. She and I both knew that she wasn't completely healed, but perhaps returning to work would become part of the healing process. She found a want ad in our local paper for a job in sales at a store within walking distance of our house! I offered to call the owner of the business to smooth the way for her, being a long-time resident in the area.

I pitched the owner on Tish's expertise, saying that she would be snatched up quickly if he didn't interview her soon. He asked her to come in the following day. George helped her write a quick résumé that night and I helped her pull together an interview outfit—it was fun for all of us, knowing that we were taking such constructive steps in the healing process.

The next day I drove Tish to the interview. She looked great, having put on a few well-deserved pounds, and she carried herself with confidence. As I sat there waiting while she was inside, I prayed for her success. Soon enough she emerged with a big smile on her face. She got the job and was to start immediately! As I predicted, she excelled at the work and had soon met many new people in our community. She was thrilled with how things were going as hope for full recovery continued to build.

Even though Tish no longer accompanied me to radiation, we continued our post radiation lunches. As we sat there one day enjoying a sandwich, she announced she felt ready to join Alcoholics Anonymous again. This was something of a milestone, a significant marker of hope, since AA is a disciplined program with a very good success rate. Tish was on a roll!

My kids were due home from college, finally having a chance to put the face to the name they had heard about during their growing up years. Easter found us all round the dining room table, with Tish as our new guest of honor, telling the funny stories of our childhood escapades.

No one understood better than Tish and I that laughter is the best medicine. We had always been cut-ups together, but now we laughed ourselves silly on many days, recalling funny stories from our childhood and acting them out. I'm sure we produced countless endorphins, aiding in our overall wellbeing.

A week later as Tishie and I sat outside on my back deck, as we did every morning while she smoked a cigarette, she told me how much she loved working with her hands in a garden. Having a decent amount of property I urged her to be my guest. Tish enlightened me on how important it is for recovering alcoholics to keep their hands busy in positive ways. She enjoyed knitting and gardening, two activities that helped her not use her hands to pick up a drink. I had never thought of it that way.

Her gardening ability would prove to be a huge help to me (and benefit to our landscape) as I was still precluded from being around too much bacteria. She also planted a pesticide-free vegetable garden that would help fortify our diminished immune systems in the warm months ahead.

Spring was in full swing now, and with it came rebirth. Tish was being reborn too, as I watched her on her days off using her hands, transforming our property. It was just what the doctor ordered!

The next step for Tish was to reconnect with her children. She had made great strides in regaining her health and it would be good for them to see how well she was doing. I encouraged her to ask her children to come for a visit, telling her they were welcome to stay with us any time. She took us up on the offer and soon her son and daughter-in-law arrived, delighted to see Tish looking so good.

Tish's daughter came next; Joanna came in for the weekend, too. As we sat around our dinner table, Joanna and Tish's daughter got acquainted. Tish reached over and patted my hand, smiling as tears of joy welled up in her eyes. It was a special moment as our daughters were getting to know one another after all these years.

Tish and her family had endured years of her illness, but all of them were finally healing, due in no small part to the gifts God provided. Patience and perseverance created the hope that always gets us through. My home was simply a sheltering space, a safe haven, where Tish could peacefully receive God's healing grace.

In the summer months that followed, Tish and I sat outside more and more. We watched as the hummingbirds went in and out of the feeders she had set up for them. The flowers she planted were in full bloom now and were a draw to the hummingbirds, as well as the beautiful butterflies that landed everywhere. It was a wonderful sight to behold. Tish had worked hard to turn our property into a Garden of Eden of sorts. I was so grateful for the beauty of nature she brought to our little piece of heaven, up high on our back deck as we enjoyed each other's company.

As usual we started talking about our kids and reminiscing about old times. She reminded me of when George was overseas in the mid-1970s, and I was back in Massachusetts with Merritt for the year. Each summer, Tish and her two children visited her extended family in our home state. Merritt was four at the time . . . as was her son. We recalled all the things we did together that precious week, including going to the drive-in movie with all three kids. It was surreal, being there with the kids when as children, we were the ones, watching the drive-in movies every summer together. We delighted in each memory.

We were both hopeful that Merritt and her son would be able to meet again one day, too, after all these years, maybe on one of their many visits to Virginia. It was a lovely thought, and we could only hope it would take place one day.

Tish's son was newly married, and she asked me when I thought Merritt would ask Karry to marry him. I said I didn't know for sure, but I knew it would happen sometime soon. Little did I know at the time, Merritt already had a plan.

A short time later, on one of Merritt's frequent calls, he said he had a few days off and was coming home, confiding to me that he planned to ask Karry to marry him in the near future. He invited George and me to accompany him for an appointment with a diamond importer. Days later, after he arrived back home, we met with the diamond experts. After

Merritt chose the perfect stone, it touched my heart when he pulled out a picture of the setting he'd seen Karry admire in a bridal magazine. The jeweler promised he would make it happen.

Merritt was excited; I was, too. Wow, my first baby getting engaged!

Months after Merritt returned to West Virginia, he called to say he had received the engagement ring, and it was just what he envisioned it to be. He was trying to surprise Karry with his proposal, but each time he planned something, she seemed suspicious. I listened, while placing the final ornaments on our beautiful artificial Christmas tree that we put up each year in the late fall. The tree was twinkling in the corner of our living room when it hit me. I excitedly said, "Merritt what about putting the ring in a box under the tree with your proposal inside? Karry would never guess you would give her the engagement ring here!"

Merritt sounded intrigued, saying that might just work. For now, it would remain our little secret.

Christmas was almost here and my family was arriving soon. George decorated the outside of our house the way I like it, my mother comparing it to Chevy Chase's movie, *Christmas Vacation*.

My extended family was excited to see Tish, too. It had been a long time since my mother and my Uncle Donnie had seen her. Thankfully, by this time she looked like her old self again. No one could have imagined what she looked like the day we first picked her up. I was so proud of all she had accomplished with each new day.

As I watched her laughing and having fun, I couldn't help but think about what a difference a year makes. I had received Tish's phone call last year on Christmas Day, after she miraculously received my rainbow letter. She was drinking herself into oblivion every night with no hope for the future. But due to God's grace and divine intervention, here she was now, whole and healthy, ready to celebrate Christmas with her old friend and her friend's family. I knew as I watched on that we both had so much to be grateful for.

On Christmas Eve, we all attended church, crowding into one pew. It was cold outside, so it seemed good to be close to each other on this holy night, praying and singing the carols. I tried keeping my emotions of gratitude in check as I looked down the long pew, seeing the faces I loved and knowing we were together once again sharing the holidays. "God is good," a phrase my mother often said, came to mind.

Early Christmas morning Merritt worked at surprising Karry. Typing up the perfect proposal, placing it in the cover of a white-quilted jewelry box that housed her ring, and placing that box into another box that he wrapped to throw her off.

After dinner everyone gathered in the living room to open Christmas gifts. As the Christmas carols played in the background, we all celebrated the special day. After almost all the gifts were given out, George snuck Karry's box under the tree without anyone noticing. Merritt made sure it was the last gift given. When Karry opened the box she burst into tears, answering yes to his question tucked into the box's cover. It was a joyful and emotional moment for all of us, and I thanked God I was still here to witness it!

At Tish's one-year anniversary of being alcohol-free, we celebrated with a special dinner and cake and ice cream. When George and I congratulated her, she shared she had nicknamed us the "Suburban Angels."

Later that evening Tish and I went to my home office to talk. She was thrilled she had reached her one-year mark and would receive her pin at AA. I reminded her of her call that Christmas Day in 1998, our first talk in years, saying, "I couldn't wait to hear back from you in January, but you never called." I hadn't quizzed Tish before about those dark days. But tonight she felt strong, wanting to tell me the whole story, admitting she never intended to call me after all. She disclosed, in fact, that she had wanted to die!

She told me about receiving my rainbow letter, saying she called on Christmas just to hear my voice one last time, to know I was all right. Then she told me about her life, saying each night on her walk home from work, she stopped to buy beer, her drink of choice. After arriving home she set five alarm clocks, placing them in strategic spots all over her small space, to go off in five-minute intervals until finally all clocks were ringing loudly, waking her from alcohol-induced slumber.

Night after night, she said, she called out to God, asking Him to end her misery and take her home, her addiction too much to endure. But for some reason, she said, sometime after the first of the year, her prayer changed; instead, she began begging God for help.

I thought about the timeframe Tish referred to, realizing it was during this time that my mother bumped into her sister. Of course it was no coincidence; it was all part of God's strategy that we couldn't recognize at the first moment, but Tish said, "When you called, out the blue, with your perfect offer, I knew it was God's plan." Amazingly, the help she so desperately needed would come from an old and trusted friend whom God now called to provide hope and a healing place. I was all too happy to be the last piece of the puzzle to drop into Tish's life, helping to turn a fractured existence into a completed picture of health.

Tish continued to live happily and healthfully with us for nearly four years. She prospered in her work and became an independent individual again, in all respects except one. She still needed transportation! A car had been out of her reach for the time being, but as always, God was good to her. One day, I had a call from my home nurse who had helped me during chemotherapy days. She had often noticed Tish walking through the neighborhood and wondered if she might like to have a car of theirs they no longer needed.

I was elated to tell Tish this news as soon as she arrived home from work. We danced around the house like kids, and then Tish called my friend to gratefully accept this generous offer. The next day I picked up the rules of the road manual from the DMV and Tish began to study. Before long she was ready to take the tests and passed with flying colors. After having her picture taken, she walked towards where I waited for her, shiny new license in hand, and smiled in pure delight.

A few days later my friend's husband came over to deliver their gift, a lovely older car in mint condition. I watched from my window as he signed over the paperwork and handed Tish the car keys, the keys to her new independence. It was quite a moment to behold!

Sometime later, Tish was ready to move on, having all the pieces in place now for a healthy new life. On the day she left, she and I backed out of my driveway at the same time. We looked over at one another, seeing who would go first, smiling at each other like we shared a secret. I knew she was thinking the same thing I was: we had come a long way!

Driving ahead of her as we left the neighborhood, I looked in my rear view mirror and thought about our growing up years in Massachusetts. In our hearts, minds, and spirits we were still those same young girls, the same friends who skipped rope, talked for hours on the phone, and told secrets all night long as we slept over at each other's house; we were even the same girls who attended the Billy Graham Crusades, rededicating our lives to Christ.

As middle-aged women we held tight to God's hand, traversing uncharted territory, trusting and believing, just as we did as children, knowing we'd come through in one piece. And we were able to give each other precious gifts in the process. Tish gave me a job to do, a job that took my mind completely off cancer and allowed me to help a dear friend in need. And my gift to her was the hope that God inspired, hope that moved her along like wind in a sail. In effect, saving her saved me, just as God planned.

I was deep in thought when we came to the crossroads. Tishie waved as her car turned in the opposite direction of mine, Divine Intervention shining down on us like the sun's rays through the clouds of life. Smiling to myself, I knew I would be forever grateful for it all!

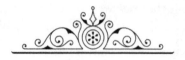

Rosana

"We'll be friends forever, won't we, Pooh?" asked Piglet.
"Even longer," Pooh answered.
A.A. Milne, *Winnie-the-Pooh*

*I*n early 1999, at one of my regular checkups, my oncologist asked if I'd be interested in counseling women who were contemplating the protocol. I was delighted and replied happily that I would help in any way I could. Weeks later my doctor called with the name of a young woman recently diagnosed who was considering the protocol. Then my doctor added, "I wanted to tell you how much she reminds us of you. She has a personality similar to yours and seems to share your belief system."

Later that day my phone rang again and Rosana introduced herself, saying she'd been to the Lombardi Center learning about the protocol and would like to know my opinion. She had a beautiful way of speaking, slowly yet intentionally, with lilts of sweetness in her voice. Never did she fully explain her diagnosis or how she found her cancer, but I knew by her consideration of the protocol that she, too, had an aggressive case. At the time she was thirty-nine.

I shared with her how pleased I was to be in the Lombardi Center's care and explained what to expect as a patient. Moreover, I emphasized how the study could benefit other women. Yet the reluctance in her voice concerned me. Naturally I wanted to pass my great experience on to another woman with the same diagnosis. The care I received at Lombardi far exceeded my expectations, and I told her so.

Continuing the hard sell, I told her about my background and how I ultimately arrived at the Lombardi Center for treatment. In telling my story I always give the glory to God, sharing the words He spoke to me as I lay on the CT scan table at Beth Israel Hospital. I told Rosana that joining the protocol made me feel I could begin the mission God gave me. I explained everything about my experience, including the CCR. She was a great listener, wanting to hear every detail. She said the doctors at Lombardi had told her of my response, and then she told me about her own spirituality; the more she talked the more I felt I'd known her all my life. She was strong yet humble, smart yet in possession of a childlike wonder at the power of God.

During our talk she said, "My prayer is, thy will be done." I admired her acceptance and encouraged her to ask God for a miracle and to believe she'd receive one. She continued to talk positively and I marveled at her spirit. Just then, while listening to her enchanting voice, my own thinking stopped. The voice of God overcame me, speaking to me once again: "Rosana will have the next CCR in the protocol." I heard His voice loud and clear, astonished that He revealed this to me, as Rosana continued to talk.

I thought momentarily about telling her, but I questioned in my mind if it was right for me to reveal God's communication to a woman whom I'd only spoken to for a little over an hour. But while thinking it over, God spoke again, this time more compellingly, giving me a clear directive, saying simply, "Tell her."

In the middle of something Rosana was saying, I interjected, "Rosana, I don't mean to interrupt you, but God spoke to me while you've been talking. He wants me to tell you that you'll have the next CCR in the protocol, urging me to tell you now." I simply blurted it out before considering her reaction. Nor did I think about the rarity of a CCR and the risk of getting her hopes up. Yet once again I trusted God's message.

Rosana didn't know me, but when I said those words, she burst out crying. I knew she wasn't crying about her circumstance; rather, she was crying because God found a way to speak to her in the midst of her crisis. I could see clearly it was an event meant to be, planned and orchestrated by the Almighty, wanting His message of hope delivered. Rosana, who was so spiritual and a true believer, could now hold onto His words as she went through the upcoming months of difficulty.

Time sped by as we continued talking for the entire afternoon, sharing our lives. She told me she was originally from Paraguay, coming to America with her family when she was a young child. She was a single, bilingual, professional woman who loved her job working with children. Instinctively I knew we'd go on this journey together. The chemistry between us was undeniable, but more importantly we shared the *Gift of Faith*.

The following week Rosana entered the protocol. I told our doctors she would have the next CCR, affirming God told me so; they listened politely, smiling at my prognosis.

Rosana and I continued to share our lives, our spirituality, and our walk, talking constantly on the phone or via e-mail. Each week found us closer than the week before, our spirits knitted together like a cozy winter sweater.

After many weeks of talking on the phone we decided to meet at a lovely restaurant in Georgetown overlooking the Potomac. We planned to meet after her appointment at the Lombardi Center. On the phone the night before, I described myself to her, giving her the color of the jacket I planned to wear. I knew oh too well that Rosana would be the woman with the hat on her head.

Spring was in the air as the sun shone brightly the day we met. Entering the restaurant we recognized each other immediately. The brim of her hat rested just above her lovely, sparkling brown eyes. To any onlooker we could have been two old college buddies meeting for lunch, embracing in our excitement of meeting face to face. We held our table by the water all day long, fascinated by our sharing and our common bond.

Rosana said chemotherapy had taken away her beautiful, long dark hair and she felt embarrassed by the way she looked. Like all of us in treatment she had also gained weight from the steroids in the chemo regimen. I responded by telling her the truth: she looked beautiful to me.

As we continued to talk I realized she had but one fear, the fear of surgery, which she had never had before, to include its scarring results. She already knew I hadn't needed a mastectomy, only a lumpectomy, and I was hopeful she'd have the same result. I also knew I could do something to alleviate her apprehension. Before leaving the restaurant, I suggested we visit the ladies' room. I told her I wanted to show her something, and finding the ladies' room empty, I turned toward her and said, "My breasts have become objects of science, and I have no problem showing you where I was cut." I asked her if she'd like to see the area, and she shook her head yes.

I undid the first few buttons of my blouse and exposed my left breast just above the nipple area, pointing to the small, undramatic scar. "That's my incision." Rosana moved in for a closer look, saying, "That's it?" I smiled at her and replied, "That's it," as I buttoned up my blouse. The expression on her face revealed how grateful she was to see the minor cut. It was obvious she was trying to compose herself when finally she said,

"I will never forget what you've done for me today." It was such a simple act, yet it relieved her mind and her fears were gone.

As we left the restaurant, soaking in the rays of the setting sun, we said our goodbyes. Our day of sharing had come to an end. Rosana was now at peace and she thanked me for my time, stepping forward to give me a big hug. At the end of our embrace we stepped back. Taking each other's hands we stood there for a moment, smiling, knowing we'd be friends forever!

As the days and weeks flew by, I wished I could meet with Rosana more often but my immune system was still not up to par. I was to stay away from crowds, especially during flu season. Rosana needed to be careful, too, as she underwent our protocol's aggressive chemotherapy, so I supported her in other ways, with an encouraging e-mail or a special card.

Late night talks were a favorite of ours. One night while talking about beloved movies, I shared mine, "The Wizard of Oz," adding "Somewhere Over The Rainbow" was my favorite song. Rosana could hardly wait to speak. "Cathy, that's unbelievable, it's my favorite song, too!" We laughed out loud at our similarities, two strangers only months before finding yet another common thread.

Neoadjuvant therapy was coming to an end for her. She had remained valiant throughout it all, never complaining. Surgery lay ahead, so we decided to meet at a restaurant the day before. I brought her a goody basket for after her operation, in which I tucked a card from my heart, writing about our friendship and how our Heavenly Father planned it in the long ago, reminding her we were old souls. I told her that God knew we were strong, we were in the same study for a reason: our doctors were learning so much from us, gathering information, finding clues to help other women and possibly finding a way to end the disease. Either way we were on a mission, and I reminded her she was the next CCR!

That night my prayers were even longer than usual and I drifted off to sleep with Rosana's name on my lips. The following afternoon I called the recovery room at the hospital, but Rosana still wasn't there. Late that night I made my last call to Georgetown; Rosana was finally in her room. A nurse picked up my call, saying Rosana's family was with her, but she wanted to speak with me for a moment. A weary Rosana came on the line and I asked her how things had gone. She said the surgeon had just left her room.

"What did he say about your surgery?" I gently asked.

Hesitant to reply, she said softly, "He felt he may have hit more cancer. He'll wait for the pathology report, but more than likely I'll need further surgery next week." We both knew what that meant: mastectomy.

I protested and explained that pathology would be the group to reveal for certain what was going on in her breast. Then I reminded her of what God had told me months earlier. Her voice lifted slightly when she said, "Oh my friend, even in my darkest hour you're here for me."

I responded, "No, Rosana, in your darkest hour God is here for you, just as He's always been. Remember to keep your faith; you've been given a miracle! Pathology's findings will prove you're the next CCR in the protocol, just as God promised!"

My message touched her as she took a deep breath, trying to keep her composure. She thanked me sweetly, her voice filled with emotion.

In closing I said I'd await her good news at the end of the week, after she received her investigative report; she promised to call me. Pressing the off button on my phone, I was drained, having given Rosana all the positive energy in my being. I lay my head back in my chair and stared at the ceiling.

I resolved to believe that no matter what was told to Rosana tonight, I would go on believing she was the next CCR in the protocol and that God would see her through; I just knew He would! Disturbed by Rosana's news, I went to tell George and found him in our bedroom choosing his suit for work the next day. After telling him what the surgeon said, George walked toward me, and taking my hands pulled me to the edge of our bed where we sat facing one another. I could see he was troubled as he revealed that he felt I'd given Rosana false hope during these months, reminding me he'd warned me of this possible outcome.

I asked, somewhat displeased, "What are you talking about?"

He continued, "You told her she was the next CCR in the protocol, she believed you, but now her surgeon thinks there's more cancer, which means she'll have a mastectomy next week."

He continued to gently lecture me. "Cathy, you just can't tell the women who call you for help that they're going to have a miracle."

Defiantly, I pulled my hands away and stood up. I said, "I revealed to Rosana what God told me to tell her and I'd do it again if He asked me to!"

George closed his eyes, shaking his head in frustration, and said, "Have it your way, but understand that Rosana is at Georgetown tonight suffering because of what you told her."

He walked away, continuing to prepare for tomorrow. I was annoyed and shaken by his comments. I didn't even say goodnight as I left our room and headed for my office sanctuary, wanting to be alone to pray and get my peace back.

Entering my space, I turned on only one light and closed the door behind me. With spiritual music playing softly in the background, I sat at my desk and began to pray. I stared at the crosses on my wall, confirming what God revealed to me months earlier, believing with all my heart Rosana was the next CCR. Tears welled up and streamed down my face as I thought of Rosana lying in her hospital bed receiving the distressing news. But I promised myself I'd not allow my faith to falter. I'd continue to hold onto the word of knowledge God gave me, waiting for His truth to be revealed.

I lay my forehead on my arms and, losing control, sobbed out loud, my heart aching for my friend. I called out to God, asking for His peace, and holiness began to fill my small refuge. Breathing it in, my spirit lifted, my convictions grew even stronger, and the peace of God encircled me.

The world would try to disprove God's exchange, but I wasn't listening to the world or its doubts.

Vowing to stay in faith, I continued to pray for Rosana. When my phone finally rang later that week, an elated Rosana called out my name. She had just met with the surgeon, who told her he had apparently hit scar tissue from the tumor bed, nothing more. He read aloud the pathology report, deeming Rosana the next CCR in the protocol!

We screamed with excitement. There would be no mastectomy for Rosana; she, too, had been given a miracle. The insight God had given me months earlier was now corroborated by science, Praise God!

During the previous months I'd told Leda all about Rosana; they hadn't met as yet, but Leda was praying for Rosana, too. After all, we were the "Women of the Protocol." I called Leda to give her the good news about Rosana's outcome. Naturally she was elated and suggested it was time to meet in person, so we all signed up for the Millennium Race for the Cure in Washington, D.C., held in June 2000.

We met at the rally the day before, where Leda and Rosana clicked immediately. The day was sweltering hot, so we went in search of a cold drink as the throng was registering. In the registration area we met a woman who had also survived inflammatory breast cancer, the type Leda had. The two of them immediately began comparing notes, and the woman shared she'd lived healthfully for the past eight years after her treatment! It had been a long, hot walk to find a cool drink, but it proved a blessing for Leda. She, who was so strong and brave, burst out crying, having been given the gift of hope by another survivor. Rosana and I were overjoyed for our friend.

Leda and Rosana were easily becoming friends on their own, and Rosana quickly nicknamed us "The Three Amigas." Then and there, we promised that one day we would have one of the largest fundraising teams in the Race for the Cure. Walking back to the festivities arm in arm, I asked my friends, "Would you like to be on TV?" I wanted to commemorate this special day forever. They were enthused, but they asked how? I said leave it to me—many networks were covering the rally.

Within minutes I had introduced myself to a reporter, explaining that we were three women in an aggressive stage III breast cancer research protocol at the Lombardi Center. I said we were all doing well and asked if he'd like to do a spot about us. He jumped at the chance, confirming that my sales ability was still intact.

The camera rolled and the reporter asked our names. I was then asked to talk about our experience and my statements flowed easily. The Lombardi Center had done such good work in the protocol that we stood there as survivors to prove it! We were shining examples of what monies raised for research can do. The interview went well and hope was everywhere. It had been an exciting and deeply memorable day.

Our son Merritt's wedding day finally arrived in March 2001. Karry, his beautiful bride, and I waited at the back of the church for our cue. The organist began playing Ave Maria as Blake, the best man, came to escort me. Merritt, looking so handsome as he stood at the altar, winked at me as I walked the center aisle.

Many of our family and friends joined in our celebration. Among the crowd I spied Rosana out of the corner of my eye; our glance told of knowing the enormity of the moment. She and I understood it well: I was healthy and whole again and by God's Grace had made it to my son's wedding! I was thankful for yet another answered prayer, and Rosana's presence made it all the sweeter.

Eight month's later when Rosana went for her regular checkup, God's intervention showed itself once again. We now shared the same oncologist, who ordered the normal CT scan as part of the protocol. All appeared to be well, but when an infinitesimal spot showed up outside the breast, the doctor ordered a PET scan and a biopsy. The doctor's tenacity resulted in the discovery of a well-hidden pre-breast cancer cell in Rosana's body, meaning she now had stage IV breast cancer. She was immediately put on Herceptin to stop any other breast cancer cells in their tracks.

Rosana accepted her new diagnosis with pure grace and faith, saying sweetly, "It's just the way it is, my friend." We never went deeply into this new medical discovery. She didn't want others to know she had stage IV breast cancer, confiding months earlier there were certain people in her life she considered to be her angels, sharing the ups and downs of this disease, and for her that was enough. She wasn't trying to hide her diagnosis; she just wanted to live her life fully, enjoying each day, instead of always talking about cancer.

As we discussed this latest development I couldn't help but remind her of everything God had done to expose this new problem, reminding her of our miracle, saying God had plans for us. Rosana was devout in her faith, already knowing all I told her, but I wanted my words to resonate in her head. She answered sweetly, "You know, my friend, you're one of my angels."

Amazingly enough, I already knew she was one of mine!

Rosana responded well to treatment, and the years passed by quickly. She was back in shape, walking regularly, and ready to travel again. She and her mother took a long-awaited holiday to their beloved Paraguay, visiting extended family. When Rosana returned, she phoned to tell me all about the trip, in particular describing two cherished mementos she had brought home. One was a beautifully carved wooden sculpture that evoked the hand of God holding a child in His palm. The other was a framed picture of the sculpture with a paraphrase of the verse from Isaiah 49:15 printed next to it: "See! I will not forget you . . . I have carved you on the palm of my hand." She told me how much the words meant to her, and that she had placed both objects on her nightstand. They comforted her just before falling off to sleep, reminding her that she was in God's loving care!

With the passage of time our lives became busier, and Rosana and I weren't able to see each other as often as we used to, so we vowed no matter what, we would meet every July at our oncologist's office. I was there for my yearly checkup and she was there for treatment. After our morning appointments we ran across the street like giddy schoolgirls to our favorite restaurant for a day of catch-up, belated birthday gifts in hand.

Rosana did well on Herceptin for six years until early July 2007, when she called to say she had had a setback, landing her in the hospital. Her drug was being changed to a new one that had just come on the market. She would lose her hair again and not feel well for a while, but she maintained her faith-filled stance.

Shortly after Rosana started the new chemo drug we met for lunch. She could eat nothing but Saltines and ginger ale and should have been home resting, but she said, "Cathy, you are the one person I'd never cancel with! Just being with you makes me feel better."

We talked and talked, exchanging gifts. I told her I would one day write the story about the two of us, reminding her that once my book was published, she'd be the poster child for stage IV breast cancer, proving you can still have a good life of family, work, travel, and friends while keeping cancer at bay! My enthusiasm made her grin and say, "You're just too cute, my friend."

After lunch her mother came to pick her up. Saying our goodbyes for now I hugged her tight as I helped her into the car. As they drove away she turned back to catch a glimpse of me, throwing me a kiss and waving sweetly.

In the New Year of 2008, Rosana had been on her new medicine for six months and was tolerating it quite well. We had decided to get together in late spring when the weather would be good, but in April, as I opened my mailbox, I found a package from Rosana. A gorgeous bracelet was enclosed along with a birthday card, on which she wrote that she knew the bracelet was meant for me the moment she saw it. The card went on to say she loved me and we'd talk soon. I was touched by her thoughtfulness but wondered why she had mailed the gift instead of waiting for our get-together. Nonetheless, I shook off my puzzlement and went out to buy a special thank-you card and told her I was looking forward to seeing her soon.

As time went on, I was surprised I hadn't heard back from her, but life, with its busyness, didn't allow me to analyze her silence too closely. When she finally did call, she asked if I'd received her gift, which meant she hadn't received my thank-you card. After I clarified my end of the story she said, "I'm at my mother's right now. She thinks she saw a card from you but she can't seem to find it."

In calm Rosana fashion she then explained that she'd recently been in the hospital due to dehydration and was recovering at her mother's after developing a problem with her blood. She never went into specifics, except that the doctors were working on it.

After finishing our talk, I began putting the puzzle pieces together. With growing dread I realized she must have septic poisoning, a dangerous problem that had taken my grandmother's life years earlier. Later that evening when I knew Rosana would be fast asleep, I called her mother, telling Livia of my suspicions, which she confirmed. I said I'd have everyone I know praying for Rosana by morning.

A week later Rosana was in the hospital having her abdomen drained. When I reached her at home that evening she said she felt more comfortable but weak. She was taking powerful antibiotics to fight the infection but said she would call me soon.

On a beautiful weekend in early June our family gathered for a barbecue. As I came back in the house to get something, the phone rang; it was Rosana, sounding like her old self. After catching up a bit, I asked how she was feeling. She said the doctors had tried every antibiotic in their arsenal and now had her on the last one remaining. Then she said very matter of factly, "You know, my friend, they say this is the end." The end of what, I pondered?

"What do you mean, Rosana?"

In her sweet, enchanting voice she said, "You know, my friend, the end!" Suddenly, my heart was in my throat, knowing she was talking about dying. I went to my office sanctuary and sat down, kicking into high-gear cheerleader mode, saying, "No matter how smart the doctors are, Rosana, they're not Almighty God," reminding her of all we had yet to accomplish.

As I ran out of encouraging words, the phone went silent. Finally Rosana took a deep breath and answered softly yet purposefully. "My friend, I feel like one of those relay runners in the Olympics—you know, the runner who gives all they have to give, then they pass the baton to the runner who is stronger and who they know can win the race." I could visualize what she was saying as she continued, "So you see, my friend, I'm passing the baton to you. You'll take it to the finish line for all of us!"

I was moved by her words as I tried to hold back my emotions, answering resolutely, "Rosana, don't give up, whatever you do!" She answered with the same words she'd repeated over and over, for nearly a decade of our friendship, "Thy will be done, my friend."

I told her I'd continue holding her up in prayer, praying that this last antibiotic would eradicate the bacteria in her body. She said she loved me and thanked me for being one of her angels. I told her I loved her, too, trying to push the thought out of my mind that this was farewell, convincing myself it wasn't.

She said she would call me next week. "Run along now, enjoy your family." As we said our goodbyes she whispered, "I'm tired, my friend, it's been a long fight."

By now my family was calling me to come eat. I started to go back out, where I could see my granddaughter, Reagan, blowing bubbles and running around to catch them. "Ma, come outside and see how big my bubbles are!" she called. As I wiped away my tears my little princess took my hand and led the way.

In the early evening a week later after I had returned from a brief trip to the grocery store, George told me Rosana's sister had called while I was out. It must have been God's providence that allowed me to be out of the house rather than take the call myself. George very tenderly told me that Rosana had passed away that morning, cushioning the blow that nonetheless felt like a left hook to my chin. I retreated to my bedroom and fell on the bed and began to pray, tears pouring down my face. As with so many other times of tribulation, I went to God.

My prayers finished, I began talking to Rosana, whispering her name into the darkness of my room, telling her what she meant to me, talking for some time until my emotions were spent. Then my mind went to our last conversation, realizing she truly called to say goodbye! In that devastating moment I called out to her, "I will sorely miss you, my friend" and pleaded with her to give me a sign that she was on the other side.

A few days later Rosana's family held a celebration of her life at a church in Maryland. A large portrait of Rosana stood on an easel, a contented smile on her pretty face as she gazed out at us. I looked over the program that outlined hymns and speakers and noticed that the last song of the service would be none other than "Somewhere Over the Rainbow." I thought of the many times she and I had discussed that one song over the years. Before the service began, Rosana's mother quietly greeted many of us in the crowd, and she told me that Rosana had requested the song herself as she thought about her last days.

I could hear her sweet voice during our late-night talks, saying, "You know, my friend, if birds fly over the rainbow, then why can't I?" I suddenly realized that her words were an affirmation, meant for those few of us she called her angels, and I knew with great joy and certainty that she meant it as her sign. Today, her message of hope was loud and clear, she was now over the rainbow, she was on the other side; she had made it! Rosana's humble acceptance of "Thy will be done" had brought her home, to a heaven lonesome for her pure heart and wondrous childlike faith.

Rosana was forty-eight when she died, nine years after her miraculous CCR. Through God's ongoing care and the expertise of her doctors, she was also able to keep stage IV breast cancer under control and to live her life abundantly. What a testament of hope and inspiration for other women!

A year after Rosana passed away I received a package from her mother. I took it to my office to open, and pulled out two bequests, gently unwrapping each of them, placing them on my desk for a closer look. The first was a large wooden hand with a child leaning into it, resting contentedly; the second was a framed print of the verse from Isaiah. I was taken aback as I marveled that of all the possessions in Rosana's home, Livia was led to give these treasured remembrances to me. Yet, I had never mentioned them to Livia before, nor discussed my and Rosana's conversation concerning them. I then read the note she enclosed: "These precious keepsakes meant so much to Rosana, and she would want you to have them." How astonishing that these spiritual souvenirs found their way to me, Divine Destiny at work.

As I came to the end of this chapter I couldn't help but recall the many wonderful memories Rosana and I shared during the years of our sacred friendship. Sitting quietly in my workspace with music playing softly in the background, I reminisced. Suddenly, as if cued to do so, Katharine McPhee's beautiful rendition of "Somewhere Over the Rainbow" began to play.

The song touched me, lifting my spirit, as I embraced the lessons Rosana passed on, understanding that time would never change the bond we shared, and I knew in my heart, as I stared at the cherished mementos on my desk, that one day we would meet again, somewhere over the rainbow!

The New Millennium,
Filled with Spirit and Grace

It is never too late to be what you might have been.
George Eliot

aving shared the stories and inspiration of my three dear
friends, I will return to my own journey now, which proceeded with several more twists and turns, but thankfully,
the worst would be over.

When Tish first came to live with us, I was entering the final stage
of the protocol, needing only to complete radiation. I had visited my
oncologist for a checkup, and as she examined me, I reminded her that
one day my book would be out there (maybe even on Oprah!), inspiring
women to live in hope and faith. Grabbing a stethoscope from a nearby

table, she smiled and said, "Whatever you say, Cathy, I have no doubt it will happen." I thought about her response, not wanting her to think because I said so it would happen. Rather, it was what God wanted, and I told her so.

Then she became serious. Taking her stethoscope she turned it sideways and gently tapped me in the middle of my bare chest, saying, "I knew what you were trying to say, but God always needs a messenger, and He chose you!" The words she spoke were profound, touching my spirit and confirming what God had planned for me.

My next appointment was a follow-up with my transplant doctor. He was pleased with my continued progress, saying I no longer needed to wear my mask outdoors and could make my appointments for radiation—this was progress!

I was warned about the possible side effects of radiation: exhaustion, nausea, and painful sunburns. Immediately after each treatment and several times a day I rubbed aloe vera over my chest, praying the soothing gel would prevent a burn. As it turned out, I sailed through radiation with no ill effects at all. Thank you, Lord!

An unforeseen benefit of my radiation treatment arose when I was able to talk with other women in the waiting room about my story of hope. The waiting room became one of the many platforms God prepared for me, platforms that would become increasingly public for the future He had in mind for me.

After my final radiation appointment that marked the end of all my cancer treatments, George wanted to commemorate the day. Driving to a local nursery, he bought a tulip tree in my honor. He brought it home and planted it carefully, preparing the ground just so and adding the right mix of nutrients. The tree was in its infancy, a small and fragile shrub. We were told it would one day be a tall, robust tree adorned with beautiful blossoms—a perfect symbol of life taking hold, with hope and faith and thriving despite all obstacles. As a glorious spring day came to an end,

George tamped the last bit of dirt around the base of this joyous addition to the middle of our front yard. Leaning on his shovel, he said assertively, "Honey, this tree signifies the end of all your treatments." It had been a long haul, but it was finally over!

Tish, who had also been working in the yard, joined us as we admired the new addition. I was in the middle and pulled them close, understanding the enormity of the moment. The warmth of the setting sun embraced us, as if God Himself was smiling down on the three of us, and all seemed right with the world.

About a year after I had surgery, when it was time for Blake to return to college, we were driving to West Virginia on a hot and humid August day. I had pulled on shorts and a short-sleeve shirt for the trip. We had hours of driving ahead of us, but we wouldn't notice, as Blake and I could talk on any subject, family or philosophical, and the talks would be deep and honest and I loved every minute of it.

As we were closing in on Huntington while solving the world's problems, I noticed Blake staring at my left arm. He interjected, "Mom, I have to tell you something."

Wondering what was so urgent, I said, "What's on your mind, son?"

In his straightforward manner he said, "Don't take this wrong, Mom, but I'm looking at your left arm and it's huge."

I looked at both arms, and he was right; my left arm was much larger than my right, alarmingly so. I didn't know what was wrong but wondered about the significance of the swelling being on the left side, since that was where the cancer had been.

As soon as I could get to a phone I called my oncologist, who urged an immediate appointment with my surgeon. She explained that the problem could be lymphedema, a serious condition, which can occur after a dissection under the arm. I said I would call the surgeon right away, but instead of getting myself upset, I stayed in faith, knowing I was healed of stage III aggressive breast cancer. A swollen arm would be the least of my worries. George joined us over the weekend, as we helped the kids settle in for a new school year, enjoying our time together. I was determined not to let this latest issue interfere with time spent with our family.

First thing Monday morning I found myself signing in at the surgeon's office, ready to hear what he had to say. After examining my left breast and arm, he was visibly upset when he said, "Unfortunately, you have lymphedema." Pushing his fingers through his thick dark hair, he lamented, "I had hoped a year after surgery that you were in the clear."

In layman's terms, lymphedema can occur after one or more lymph nodes have been removed. If the remaining lymph nodes can't compensate for the loss, the infection-fighting fluid normally circulating through lymph nodes and lymph vessels can't drain properly, resulting in blockage and swelling. Left untreated, lymphedema causes serious complications, including chronic pain, cellulitis, and hardening and thickening of the skin.

The surgeon immediately sent me to a physical therapist to begin the process of reducing the swelling. The therapist taught me to wrap my arm to push the fluid back into my body and also gave me exercises to do, encouraging me to swim whenever possible, all in an effort to keep my arm healthy. After several weeks of therapy my left arm was still larger than my right, but it was starting to look more normal.

I then needed to be fitted for a compression sleeve, which was accomplished after taking careful measurements along the length of my arm. I will wear a sleeve for the rest of my life, but I consider this a small price to pay for my life being spared! The sleeve feels like a second skin to me now and is really not very noticeable—it's just another adversity I've moved beyond as I remain in God's healing grace.

I've mentioned public platforms God has prepared for me so that my message of hope and inspiration will reach as many women as possible. Two other platforms of note included an interview on the *QVC* network during Breast Cancer Awareness Month in October 1999 and a subsequent article in my hometown newspaper.

The *QVC* network had selected the Lombardi Center of Georgetown University Hospital as one of the beneficiaries of fundraising efforts of the annual Fashion Footwear Association of New York (FFaNY) Shoes on Sale for innovative breast cancer research. To my pleasant surprise Georgetown asked me to be interviewed for a segment *QVC* would broadcast throughout the upcoming three-hour gala special. The interview took place in the hospital, where I talked about what the research protocol meant to me, demonstrating how research money was being used to save women's lives. For my part I had but one request: would *QVC* mention I was writing a book about my remarkable recovery?

After the *QVC* interview, I decided to write an article for my hometown paper, the Duxbury Clipper. My mother had owned a gift store in the center of town, where many of the townspeople shopped and had known me since I was a child. During the years George and I traveled abroad they often asked, "How's Duxbury's Hometown Girl and where is she now?" That sweet saying stuck in my head. In the article I told everyone how I was doing and thanked them for their prayers, then talked about the *QVC* special, where they might catch a glimpse of me. The paper published my article, again providing a way for women to know that hope is paramount.

The *QVC* fundraiser was a great success and at the end of the show, as requested, the host mentioned I was writing a book and wished me well.

I was grateful for this message of hope and for reaching the multitudes of viewers who were concerned about breast cancer.

In late November 1999, I took out the Christmas decorations. While opening one of the boxes, I found the letter I had written to myself almost a year earlier, tucked under an angel. I opened it eagerly, and just as my letter predicted, I was now on the other side of the mountain, looking forward to each new day, believing in my purpose, writing the outline for my book: the book God told me to write!

For ten years after I first became a cancer patient I continued to have regular, frequent checkups, with a few changes in doctors. My beloved oncologist, who had seen me through so much and had treated me so brilliantly, moved on to the Midwest after receiving a prestigious award to continue to develop new research ideas for treating breast cancer. She shared that my tissue sample was one of the contributing factors in winning the award. I was elated, praising her success. I couldn't help but think how God had orchestrated our alliance, His Divine plan at work.

My new oncologist, a man who also treated Rosana, continued my excellent and compassionate care. When we first met, he asked me to tell him my story. I warned him it was a long one, but he appeared interested, leaning back in his chair and folding his hands in front of him. The most important part of my story is always that God spoke to me, giving me a miracle! At my story's end the doctor smiled and said, "That's just wonderful," and that's when I recognized that he was a spiritual man, too. He said, "You know, Cathy, we professionals need to hear inspirational stories such as yours, giving us hope as well."

The doctor put me on a three-month schedule of checkups, which eventually stretched to six months and then yearly as my health remained exceptional. Finally, in 2008, ten years after my breast cancer diagnosis, my oncologist said, "Cathy, this should be your last appointment with me, unless of course you have a question or a problem. You've been cancer-free for ten years now, and when you leave my office today, statistically speaking, you're just like any other woman walking around on the streets below regarding breast cancer."

Then he explained that after ten years without a recurrence, the medical community considers one cured. This came as a shock to me as I had no idea I'd ever be dismissed from oncology. I never questioned or delved into reasons for future appointments with my doctors, I simply trusted God.

Over the years I had grown very fond of this brilliant doctor, not just as a professional but also as a person, and I told him so. He smiled at me and then patted my shoulder and left the room, bidding me good day. I was healed; sick people needed his attention.

Still somewhat stunned I walked to the window and pulled back the sheers, peering out at the view from the thirteenth floor. I stood there admiring the cloudless sky as I mused I'd been discharged from oncology! Looking across the street I could see shadows of people going to and fro in other buildings. The world outside was busy in its usual way, yet I had just been told something no one else knew: I'd come full circle! Just to think I was back to being like any other woman on the streets below was awe-inspiring.

Leaving the building, I pulled my purse strap over my left shoulder as the sun warmed my skin. I thought of the gift of faith God had given me, allowing me to entrust my life to Him, my future always in His hands. Gratitude flooded my heart and mind as tears of joy welled up, and in that sweet, spirit-filled moment I recalled my father's words.

"Yes, Daddy," I whispered, my voice filled with emotion, "You were right all along . . . all you have to do is have faith."

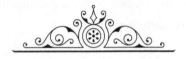

Epilogue

There are only two ways to live your life. One is as though nothing is a miracle. The other is as though everything is a miracle.

Albert Einstein

In 1998, my treatment for aggressive stage III breast cancer was cutting edge; today it's considered standard treatment, based on research done in protocols like mine, making life expectancy completely different today. To think I may have contributed to this advancement brings me great joy.

In 2009, I went ahead with the plans Leda, Rosana, and I made to have one of the largest fundraising teams in the Susan G. Komen Global Race for the Cure® in Washington, D.C., naming our team "The Three Amigas," Rosana's nickname for our friendship. Livia and Maria, Rosana's mother and sister, worked tirelessly in this effort, along with Leda's daughter and step-daughter, who traveled to Washington to walk with us in the race. Family and friends along with all the people they knew and we knew got involved. We met our goal and were one of the top fundraising teams, raising almost $20,000! I could almost see Leda and Rosana walking with us, the two of them smiling arm and arm, Rosana saying, "You're just too cute, my friend!"

In the busyness of life I was remiss in keeping in touch with my oncologist from the protocol, but in the fall of 2009 my opportunity arose. One of our local television news channels, WUSA, was preparing a mini-series about breast cancer and wanted to include a piece about me called "One Woman's Miracle," anchored by Andrea Roane, who created the Buddy Check 9 program for breast cancer awareness. To prepare for my interview I decided to call my oncologist and catch up with her after so long. She was delighted to hear from me! After chatting a bit I mentioned that I had already told Andrea about my CCR, the Complete Clinical Recovery But the doctor corrected me. "You mean Complete Clinical Response," she said.

I replied, "I thought it stood for Complete Clinical Recovery?"

"No, it stands for Response," she repeated.

We finished our conversation, promising to get together in the near future. I turned my desk chair toward the window, taking in the beautiful fall day outside. My view was somewhat obscured by the tulip tree planted eleven years earlier to mark my recovery, having grown two stories high since I completed treatment.

Thinking back on our conversation in 1998, I sat there contemplating the doctor's words, certain that she had said Complete Clinical Recovery, when in actuality she had said Complete Clinical Response.

I recalled praying daily for a Complete Clinical Recovery. To me those words meant I had a spontaneous healing through God's Grace and medical science; I was cured of breast cancer. To my doctor, the words meant that she was learning remarkable things from my experience as the first patient in the protocol to achieve a CCR. Her research on my tissue samples would go on to help countless other women. It took eleven years for the subject to come up again and for me to learn that my doctor and I were off by one word, but the meaning of that word was crucial to each of us. Almighty God in His infinite wisdom had given both of us what we asked for!

The day of my interview, I met Andrea in the lobby of the Lombardi Center. She was lovely and made me feel completely at ease. The cameras started to roll, and I couldn't help but think how far I'd come, from my initial frightening diagnosis to the healing I was given, to the spiritual growth I'd experienced. And here I was once again, telling my story, fulfilling God's plan for me.

Just then the Lombardi Center's Director of Oncology entered the room, followed by his entourage of students. Andrea, a seasoned interviewer, cut to the chase and asked if in fact I had a miracle in 1998. I was on the other side of the room, waiting to hear his response.

Without hesitation he replied, "A miracle from a variety of sources, but truly a miracle." It was a beautiful moment to behold.

In reflecting on the past number of years, it's clear that George and I survived all that life dealt us as we stayed in the day, believing God would take us through—and He did. In our years of adversity, we grew stronger, making our family bond even tighter than before. I have sat at our children's college graduations, weddings, and welcomed their babies into our family, thanking God for it all, including for my life, prayers answered, and for the moment.

Merritt stayed in West Virginia to be with his girlfriend, Karry, and to see the kids though their remaining college years, as he promised. During Merritt's time at the bank, he won many awards for his achievements there, but in time he moved on to medical sales and became a big success in the biotech industry. He and Karry recently celebrated twenty years of marriage. They are a great couple and their union has given us two precious grandchildren—our beautiful Reagan and our handsome grandson, Drake. They live in Roanoke, Virginia, about three hours away from us. The school where they attend has given Reagan and Drake a wonderful education and a strong Christian foundation that compliments Merritt and Karry's parenting. We are very proud of all of them.

Blake returned home after earning his master's degree. He married shortly thereafter and had two beautiful little girls, Lynleigh and Brynn. His marriage proved difficult at best and ended in divorce. Blake worried he had missed his happily ever after. I assured him that his meant to be was still out there looking for him, too! And that we would continue to stay in faith and prayerfully, it would happen.

One day, a beautiful girl—inside and out—named Andrea Gess stepped into Blake's life. Andrea, a devout Christian, had never been married before and longed for children of her own. She fell madly in love with Blake and his precious daughters. A few years later, they had a gorgeous wedding, and the following year, they welcomed their sweet little miracle baby girl, Blakely, into the family. We feel blessed to have Blake and his family living only five minutes from our front door.

Our sweet Joanna climbed the ladder of success in the business world in the Washington, D.C. Metropolitan area. We are so proud of all she has accomplished thus far in her life. And while working hard, she met and fell in love with a wonderful guy named Grant. He nicknamed Joanna "Snugs" (short for snuggles). We have so enjoyed seeing their relationship grow over these past few years. They have so much in common and are so right for each other. Throughout these many years, Joanna continued to save Sundays for family day, and where Blake and his family join in as well, my grandmother's tradition lives on.

My sweet Uncle Donnie has naturally grown older with the passage of time, but he continues his tradition of calling me on my birthday, serenading me to "Let me call you sweetheart." His voice doesn't quite hold the tune like it used to, but with each passing year I cherish his loving rendition even more.

Katy left the company we worked for not long after me. She asked me to pick her up on her last day, giving me a high five. Getting into my car, we two old friends drove off into the sunset and never looked back. Katy, who always loved children, took a chance on herself and started a home daycare.

But if there were one person I wish I could share this book with, it would be my mother. She had cheered me on throughout my diagnosis, healing, and my years of writing. Unfortunately, in 2008, she was diagnosed with a rare and deadly brain disease and was given two years to live. We immediately made plans for her to come live with us while she still possessed many of her faculties. During the first year she was in rapid decline yet still cognizant. At times, as she sat with me in my home office while I wrote, she would stare into space, and then out of nowhere would say with a smile, "That book is going to save your life," before quickly retreating into her own world.

A year later, as she was losing her battle to the insidious disease, somehow, from time to time, she still managed to get those same words out. I often wondered if it was a message she was given to impart to me. She was the matriarch of our family, and when she passed away in 2010, we knew we had lost our guiding light and our chief maker of memories. Gone would be the wonderful Christmases that she made so magical, and the hilarious stories she acted out at family gatherings. A chapter in our family's lives was forever closed.

Not a day goes by that I don't think of my mother and miss her. But now that my work is complete, I've come to realize how well she knew me. She knew that helping others through this book would also give me a new life in all respects. She wanted to encourage me the best she could as she had done many times throughout my life. But it was her parting message that gave me reason to pause and reflect. And as I do so, the summation of the past twenty-three years helps me clearly see God's intention in my life, acknowledging that His given purpose did ultimately save me! I am reminded of a favorite old hymn, "Trust and obey, for there's no other way."

My mission in writing this book has been to give hope to the hopeless and to inspire people who face great adversity, whether from cancer or other travails. I pray I've achieved that.

One day, as Katy and I enjoyed a day of friendship, she remarked, "Cath, you went through so much. God really tested you." She said this with great sadness and wished I'd never had to go through it at all.

Without hesitation I answered, "No, Katy, God didn't test me, He already knew I had a powerful faith. In 1998, He allowed me to know I'd be fine, telling me I'd go on to write a book of hope. I believed His words, knowing He chose me for this reason. So you see, without all that happened during these years of adversity, there would be no story to tell. There would only be one chapter about a miracle and that wouldn't fill an entire book!"

It has been in these years of writing and reliving my journey that I've been able to see clearly God's hand in all the days of my life. That's where feelings of love and gratitude overwhelm me. And it's in those spiritual moments, in my sweet sanctuary, and even now as I come to the end of my composing, that I imagine meeting God face to face one day, hearing Him say, "You have done well, my good and faithful servant," and I am transformed, overjoyed to have fulfilled my given purpose, my spirit uplifted forevermore!

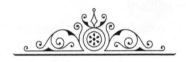

Acknowledgments. Personal Thanks. and Prayers

I've learned that people will forget what you said, people will forget what you did, but people will never forget how you made them feel.
Maya Angelou

Doctors, Nurses, and Staff

I would like to pay tribute to Dr. Roger Lange, an exceptional oncologist, formerly of Beth Israel Hospital in Boston, MA. Sadly, Dr. Lange passed away during the time of my writing, but I was privileged to meet him shortly after my diagnosis at my second opinion. He was uniquely uplifting and the first to offer me hope. To a cancer patient, hope is everything! Many years later, when my mother was undergoing a routine test, I went to see Dr. Lange. On a busy day at his office, five years after my treatment, Dr. Lange and I met face to face once again. I was finally able to express how much his words of hope and inspiration meant to me. I knew God had sent me to him for just that reason. And I am sure he is honored in God's kingdom for being one of His great healers here on Earth.

At the Lombardi Research Center at Georgetown Hospital I met Dr. Vered Stearns, the oncologist who developed the specialized aggressive stage III protocol that I would become a part of. Vered, as she asked me to call her, is an incredible woman in many ways. We developed an instant rapport, a friendship. Her genius, combined with her winning, kind, and compassionate personality, took us both on a road to discovery and healing. Mere words could never fully express my true and heartfelt gratitude to you, Vered, for being there just when I needed you most, helping to save my life through medical science, just as God planned. Vered continues her research as Co-Director of the Johns Hopkins Kimmel Cancer Center's Breast Cancer Program.

Dr. Theodore Tsangaris, M.D., was one outstanding breast surgeon. When I first met Ted as part of the protocol, I knew I was in the best of care. He made me feel so comfortable, as if we had known each other for many years. I trusted him implicitly! He is presently Chief Medical Officer and VP of Medical Affairs at Calvert Health Medical Center, Prince Frederick, MD. I will forever be grateful that God placed me in the skilled hands of Dr. Tsangaris!

Dr. Frederick Smith of Chevy Chase, MD, my longtime oncologist, is a man of healing: a brilliant, kind, and caring man. Being in the care of someone so exceptional yet down to earth gives a patient true comfort. Thank you, Dr. Smith, for your excellent care and for continuing to help so many people every day. You are a true blessing!

Dr. Reena Jha, Professor of Radiology and Surgery at Georgetown University Hospital in Washington, D.C., was someone I could always count on. During my years in the protocol she gave me the results of my scans right away after personally analyzing them. After telling her about my miracle, she took a personal interest in me, like family, she told me. Each year at my annual exams she was always relieved when the scans proved my continued good health. I will never forget her dedication. Thank you, Dr. Jha, for being a brilliant radiologist and for the beautiful person you are, inside and out.

Dr. Rebecca Zuurbier, Radiologist, is an expert in the field of breast imaging and diagnosis. We met at Lombardi where she was the Director of the Betty Lou Ourisman Breast Health Center at Georgetown University Hospital. For many years, at my annual mammogram, Dr Zuurbier scrutinized my images with her highly trained and keen eyes. Named to "America's Top Radiologists," Dr. Zuurbier is now an associate professor of Radiology and Director of Breast Imaging at Dartmouth Hitchcock Center, Lebanon, New Hampshire. Dr. Zuurbier, I want you to know what a great source of comfort you were to me as well as the many other women who entrust their lives to you daily.

Jenny Crawford, the research nurse in the protocol, was beloved by all, an angel on my path to healing. There was never a question or a task too small that Jenny didn't attend to in the most pleasant and uplifting manner. She and I kept in touch throughout my years in the research protocol, until my yearly assessment was no longer required. Jenny, I want to thank you for your dedication to cancer research and for always being ready to help in any way you could.

I would be remiss if I did not thank Jane Fall-Dickson, RN, PhD, AOCN, of Georgetown University Hospital, for her dedicated research and dissertation into the debilitating effects of stomatitis (ulcerated sores of the mouth) on breast cancer patients undergoing stem cell transplant. She began her research career focusing on the oral condition and its related pain, experienced by women and men alike, who battle the harshness of cancer treatment.

The doctors, nurses, lab technicians, receptionists, and all other hospital workers at the Lombardi Comprehensive Cancer Center and Georgetown Hospital were just amazing! Their professionalism, support, and caring, coupled with highly skilled doctors, was a win-win for me. There are no words to adequately convey my sincere gratitude and appreciation for the excellent care I received at Lombardi and for the smiles, encouragement, and spiritual essence that reside in Georgetown Hospital. After all, that's where God sent me to receive my miracle!

Family

I am so very grateful for my husband, George, and his support throughout our lives, whether it was while I was pregnant, going through childbirth, raising children, or fighting cancer. George was up for the task, and he was there for me through it all. I will never forget how he took care of me while I went through one cancer treatment after another. He went with me to every appointment and was my advocate when I needed one. *Stay in the day* was our mantra, and if ever I questioned anything, George was there to remind me that we were going to *stay in the day*. George always believed in me. He felt I could accomplish anything. Throughout these years of writing, as I burned the candle at both ends and persevered, never having written a book before, it was my husband, George, who was certain I could complete my task, believing that God chose the right person for the job. George, you will always be my high school boyfriend, my best friend, my sparring partner, my greatest supporter, and the person who never allows me to be weak. Simply put, I love you today and always, "Until the Twelfth of Never."

I was blessed with three wonderful children, Merritt, Blake, and Joanna. Since we always lived far from our extended family in Massachusetts, I made sure to emphasize the importance of our family connection. I could never have imagined that I would be diagnosed with an advanced stage of breast cancer just as my kids were college-aged. Yet as a mother, during that time, I saw the goodness in each of my kids and how they dealt with my problem.

Merritt naturally stepped up to the plate and was there for all of us. He had always been a great role model for his brother and sister and helped in every way he could. He continued to be very protective over me, calling regularly and making the long drive back home from West Virginia to spend time with me—something he did quite often. I always treasure our time together. As always, he was encouraging and cheered me on to victory on a daily basis. And I will never forget how, as a young man, he worked to help his father and I acquire our much-needed transportation! Amazing!!

Blake returned home from college every summer during those years, and we spent quality time together. We went to the movies, enjoyed backyard barbecues, and had lots of heartfelt talks about life. Blake always believed in me and admired my faith, always checking up on me and believing I would beat cancer! On days that I didn't feel completely myself, Blake would lie on my big bed with me while together we caught up on the latest "Jerry Springer Show," laughing ourselves silly. Laughter, after all, is the best medicine, and Blake's infectious laugh could always get both of us going.

Joanna, my sweet girl, took care of me the second half of her senior year in high school as I endured aggressive chemotherapy. Each day after school, she made sure to check on me and pick up my favorite smoothie. I'm sure her senior year didn't turn out the way she planned. Yet, she never complained. She stayed home with me most of the time, rather than going out with her friends, as she and her father saw me through many a rough day. Together we watched our share of the "Oprah Winfrey Show" and talked for hours on varied subjects. She helped to keep my mind occupied with her youth and differing opinions. Joanna was my companion, nurse, caretaker, encourager, and she believed in my miracle, too.

Gratitude and love could never completely describe how I feel about my children. We certainly went down some dark and scary roads together. But through our love, faith, and family devotion, we grew tighter. We learned we could get through anything together, even cancer! My children have been some of my greatest supporters and enthusiasts, believing that I would see this project through and accomplish the vision that God gave me all those years ago. Kids, I am so proud of all of you, and I feel truly blessed to be your mother. Know I'll love you forever.

Our lovely daughter-in-laws, Karry and Andrea, have each played important roles in my life, as well. We are thankful for the wonderful women our sons have chosen in this life. We feel blessed to have them in our family.

Karry, Merritt's girlfriend at the time, was on the ride with us, too. She was so thoughtful and called often to check up on me or to send a card with a sweet and uplifting message. It comforted me to know that Karry was there for the "kids" (Blake and Joanna) out at school, as well, since I was far away and going through harsh and aggressive chemotherapies. But it was when Joanna needed a co-signer for her student loan, as our credit was so negatively impacted, that Karry proved to be a true family member. Karry, saved the day by immediately stepping up to co-sign Joanna's student loan, which allowed Joanna to continue her education. That selfless act will permanently live in my heart and mind. Karry is a wonderful wife, mother, and friend to our son Merritt.

Andrea came into our son Blake's life just when he needed her most. Blake was exhausted, worn out from fighting with everything he had to gain custody of his girls. He is always striving to give his children the best life. Andrea, the consummate cheerleader, is full of love and as a devout Christian, her soothing and uplifting ways have given my son and his daughters a new life in every sense of the word. I am so grateful to have her as part of our family and with them living only five minutes away, I was able to go through Andrea's pregnancy with her and welcome the newest member of the Davis family, precious baby, Blakely.

My sweet grandchildren, Reagan, Drake, Lynleigh, Brynn, and Blakely are excited to see their names in print (well, maybe not the baby). Remarkably, they were each an answer to my fervent prayers in 1998, blessing my life in ways they will never truly understand. My hope is that my book will set an example for their generation, that when God gives you a job to do, you must see it through. As I see it, *Myrcles* is my personal legacy to each one of them and will be so for many generations yet to come. Always remember, dearest ones, that Ma loves you so very much.

My mother was always my cheerleader, believing I could do anything I set my mind to. She played a significant role in encouraging me as I wrote this book. She loved to hear what I had written, nurturing me every step of the way, believing in God's purpose for my life. But toward the end of her life, a diagnosis of Lewy Body dementia robbed her of her thoughts and sight. She needed twenty-four-hour-a-day care and was placed in a beautiful nursing facility in Cape Cod. With her brain failing her, I made the long trek to Massachusetts every six weeks to be with her and comfort her until she passed away. It was almost Christmas and the thought of leaving my mother behind was more than difficult. But I needed to get on the road to celebrate with my kids and grandchildren back in Virginia. My mother knew I was leaving as we held each other tight one last time. She had a moment of clarity as she clutched my hand and asked sweetly, "How will I think of you, Cathy, when you are gone?" I suggested she think of me at my home with my children, gathered round the Christmas tree and enjoying our favorite time of year. She shook her head sadly, closed her eyes and said, "Oh, no! I can't think of you like that!" I instantly realized how difficult that would be after all the wonderful Christmases we had shared together. Then I thought of my book and how she enjoyed being with me as I wrote it. Her grip got tighter, not wanting me to leave. I then suggested she think of me at my desk, spiritual music playing softly in the background, as God gave me the words to type. The thought of that made her smile. She lovingly lifted my hand to her lips, closed her eyes again, and kissed my hand, "Yes, dear, that's just how I'll think of you from now on." My mother's love and support, until she went to Heaven, was immeasurable! I miss you so much, Mom, and I will love you forever.

So many people wish they had sisters. My own mother was one of those people. Since I was the oldest, my mother often told me how important my sisters, Holly and Nancy, would be in my life. Years later, when we were all grown up, we left our home one by one. We left our sweet family unit and the girl's dormitory we shared in our house by the sea—the large room we played school in, where we created fairylands, watched Shirley Temple movies, anxiously awaited Santa's arrival, and whispered to each other in the darkness. Our days of swimming and playing at the beach had come to an end, or so we thought. A little more than two years ago, I was getting ready to celebrate a milestone birthday, which many doctors predicted would never happen. Holly surprised Nancy and me with an all-expenses-paid trip to Bermuda. Holly planned every detail of the fabulous trip from the invitation letter six months earlier to the crossword puzzle we had to solve to discover our destination. The time came to meet as the three sisters flew to Bermuda. Their plane from Massachusetts was filled with many friendly Bostonians, so they shared with many around them our reunion plans and the big birthday celebration ahead. We sisters planned to meet at the baggage claim area once we all arrived from our home airports. The minute we spied each other, our excitement was palpable to everyone on their flight, and they cheered at our delight.

After arriving at the beautiful hotel, our large and spacious suite was fit for queens. We were definitely spoiled being on the concierge floor with waiters who were assigned to make us happy. While we were in Bermuda we shopped, ate fabulous food, went sightseeing, shared secrets, took turns scratching each other's backs, sun bathed, and swam in the beautiful bluish-green waters. It was wonderful to just be sisters again, all by ourselves—to reminisce and enjoy each other's company as grown women. At our last night's dinner on the beach, with sand in our shoes and as the salt air cooled us off, we toasted each other and thanked Holly for the trip of a lifetime. The candles on the table lit up my sisters' smiling faces as I remembered my mother's words from long ago. Yes, we were sisters, the Alves girls in fact, grateful for each other, celebrating our connection, honoring a notable birthday, and thankful for the storms we had weathered together.

My sisters, Holly Alves Anacone and Nancy Alves Brown, are always there for me whenever I need to talk. They have listened to the stories in this book many times over, all the while, spurring me on with perfect words of love and encouragement with each new chapter of the book I finished. And they have delighted in each birthday I've been blessed to celebrate, twenty-three more since my frightening diagnosis, their support of me making my book into a reality has helped me stay on course. I love my sistahs (as we sometimes pronounce it in Massachusetts) with all my heart! And I have so appreciated their unending love and support for this vocation.

I would also like to offer a heartfelt thank you to my brother-in-law, Robert Anacone. Robert was my childhood friend and really, more like a brother to me. In 1998, he was able to get me the appointments I needed with the top oncologists in Boston immediately after my diagnosis. That intervention pointed me toward Lombardi Research Center at Georgetown University Hospital, where I would ultimately receive my miracle! I love you Rob, and I am so proud of all you have accomplished in your life!

My grandmother, Nana as I called her, was born a MacKenzie. She had four siblings who enhanced our lives with many cousins. After writing the first chapter of this book, I was asked to read it at a MacKenzie cousin reunion. When I was finished reading my cousins sang my praises, urging me on in this mission, commending my work and remaining steadfast in their love and support throughout these many years. May the good Lord continue to watch over and bless the MacKenzie Clan, keeping us close in spirit, forever enriching our lives through His loving care.

Inspirational Voices

Over these many years of writing, spiritual leaders have inspired me to be able to accomplish the task that God set before me—people such as Mother Teresa, Reverend Billy Graham, Reverend Robert H. Schuller, Reverend Pat Robertson, Dr. Norman Vincent Peale, and Joel Osteen to name a few. Positive and uplifting leaders of our time, such as Oprah Winfrey, Dr. Bernie Siegel, Tony Robbins, Deepak Chopra, and Dr. Wayne Dyer made me realize that I could do it. My thanks to all of them for their books, tapes, talks, and words of encouragement, instilling in me a "can do spirit."

Publisher and Editor

Next, I want to thank my publisher, Morgan James Publishing, for seeing my vision and understanding the impact this book has and will continue to have on people all over the world. Thank you to my editor, Susan Nelowet. The help and suggestions she offered me for my original manuscript were nothing less than exceptional. My sincere gratitude goes out to Cortney Donelson for all her help in editing the new content in my book.

Family, Friends, and Strangers Too!

I would like to thank everyone who offered up prayers on my behalf during my treatment, healing, and years of writing. You were all part of my miracle, and I will never forget your devotion.

Friends

I have been truly blessed throughout my life with wonderful friends. I subscribe to the quote, "Friends are the family you choose for yourself." Whether the friendships started when I was a young child growing up in my beloved Duxbury or during my travels as an adult, friendships have always meant a lot to me, and I think of those people as family.

I would like to thank all of you, whether near or far, for your continuous support and encouragement of this project. You have remained unwavering, always excited to hear an overview of my latest chapter and all the while cheering me on from the sidelines.

My New Friend

I will not soon forget the special stranger who came into my life from across the country, at the perfect time, predestined by God, giving me the gift of his talented photography for the cover of this book. I am deeply touched and grateful to Cinematographer Matt Herriger of Herriger Films for the beautiful photograph of Duxbury Beach. Amazingly enough, as I would soon learn, it was the beach of both our youth!

Lord Jesus, as I come to the end of my acknowledgments with my book now complete, I am reminded of my high school graduation in the 1960s when our choir sang *The Impossible Dream*. I stood there in my white cap and gown, wondering what dream you had in store for me while the words of the song touched my spirit, filling me with great emotion. Back then I could never have envisioned the path I was to take, never mind that I would be asked to write a book about it, a story that would touch other souls. But during these years I have come to realize that I have truly lived the words of *The Impossible Dream* and have been true to this glorious quest, and why the words rang true to me all those years ago. I have fought the unbeatable foe, but it was only through your love and intervention that I was able to run where the brave dare not go, hopeful that the world will be better for this, and with my miracle in place and my book set to print, I have reached the unreachable star!

Amen.

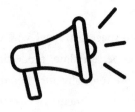

Call to Action

Dear Reader,

Thank you so much for choosing my book, *Myrcles*. My hope is that *Myrcles* has touched your life in a profound way. I pray it has showed you how to overcome adversity and *stay in the day.*

I cherish your feedback, and I would be honored if you would review my book online. In fact, one study reported that 84 percent of people trust online reviews as much as they trust their friends' opinions. Not to mention, reviews are the secret sauce that move a book up in the pages of Amazon. The more reviews authors receive on Amazon, the more exposure they get on that site. In that way, others who are searching for hope and inspiration will be able to find the book more easily. The same can be said for all our favorite bookstores and platforms, such as Barnes and Noble and GoodReads. I would so appreciate your review at any or all of these locations.

And if you enjoyed *Myrcles* as much as I hope you have, I would like to ask you to spread the word about *Myrcles* availability. You can do this by telling your family, friends, neighbors, book clubs, church groups, co-workers, Facebook page, etc. about *Myrcles*. God wanted the book to touch *countless others* so I'm asking for your help today. So many people just need a lift and a new way of thinking. *Myrcles* has already changed many lives out there. My prayer is for *Myrcles* to continue to give others hope for a better tomorrow.

I also welcome you to follow me on my *Myrcles* Facebook page, my personal page, Cathy Alves Davis, and my closed breast cancer page, Breast Cancer-Myrcles, Hope and Inspiration. Also on my Instagram account @cathyalvesdavis.

I want to let you know that I speak at all sorts of venues, and I actually attend book clubs where *Myrcles* is the book of the month. And I personally sign all attendees' books. You can also follow what *Myrcles* is up to on my website www.myrcles.com. In that way, if time permits and I am in your area, I can be part of your book club or speak to your group.

If you need a prayer, you can always reach out to me on my email, cathydavis33@gmail.com or send me a message on my Facebook pages. Know I am here for you and that I am cheering you on, no matter what you are facing.

Remember, keep believing and always look up!

Your Friend in Christ,

Cathy Alves Davis

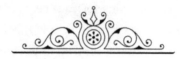

Discussion Questions

1. What is the major theme or message of the book? How can the message assist you in finding your own purpose?

2. The writer believes in "staying in the day" in all situations. Did you find this to be good advice? Do you see ways in which "staying in the day" would be helpful to you or others?

3. Is the book clearly written? How would you describe the author's style (for example, formal, conversational, academic, humorous, thoughtful, etc.)? Is the style effective and appropriate for the topic?

4. Is the author's treatment of the subject convincing? How does the author achieve credibility?

5. Does this book cause you to think about your relationships with other people in new or different ways?

6. What did you learn about the nature of adversity? Does this book contain solutions that are likely to be effective for dealing with life's challenges?

7. Which sections or passages of the book did you find especially effective or memorable?

8. How would you describe or summarize the main message of this book to someone who might be interested in it? How would you try to encourage someone to read it who might not be interested at first?

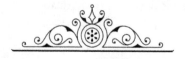

About the Author

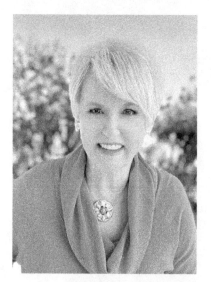

*C*athy Alves Davis is the CEO of MYRCLES, LLC. She is an inspirational speaker, author, and part-time life coach.

Cathy grew up in Duxbury, Massachusetts. She attended Bridgewater University in her home state of Massachusetts. She married her high school sweetheart, George. Together they traveled the world as George served as an officer in the United States Marine Corps. They finally settled in Montclair, Virginia and raised their family. Later this year, they will celebrate their fifty-third wedding anniversary. They have three children and five grandchildren.

In 1998, Cathy faced a life-threatening, stage III, aggressive breast cancer. At the time of her diagnosis, she was offered little hope of surviving, but Cathy had an unwavering faith in God. She volunteered to be part of a rigorous and cutting-edge research protocol at Lombardi Cancer Research Center at Georgetown University Hospital. The research results were nothing less than miraculous!! The findings proved to be a great advancement in the fight against aggressive breast cancer. The specialized protocol is now standard treatment, saving tens of thousands of women's lives to date.

For more than two decades now, Cathy has counseled, encouraged, and given hope to women everywhere. Cathy has appeared on *QVC*, "Nightline," and the *ABC* and *NBC* news. Cathy also wrote a feature story for *Breast Cancer Wellness* Magazine titled "Stay In The Day." And Cathy was featured in an article in *PWC Living* Magazine called "Finding Strength and Inspiration in 'Myrcles,'" written by Emma Young.

Cathy's testimony to the power of faith, along with excellent medical care, is revealed in *Myrcles*. *Myrcles*, spelled MYRCLES—or my miracles or your miracles—receives consistent five-star reviews!